KOMBUCHA: TEA MUSHROOM

THE ESSENTIAL GUIDE

by Christopher Hobbs

D1550577

Botanica Press
Santa Cruz, CA

Author's Disclaimer

The following information is for educational and health-increasing use only and not meant to be a prescription for any disease. If you are experiencing symptoms, I always recommend contacting a qualified health practitioner or physician for a diagnosis and total health and herbal program.

Our Commitment

We at Botanica Press are dedicated in our personal and professional lives to environmental awareness. We are strongly committed to recycling, and we gladly contribute a portion of our profits to the Nature Conservancy and other conservation groups. This book is printed on recycled paper with a minimum of 10% post-consumer waste, and the entire text is printed using soy-based ink.

♲ This book is printed on Simpson 60lb recycled paper using soy-based ink.

Other Books in the "HERBS AND HEALTH" Series

By Christopher Hobbs

Echinacea, The Immune Herb

Foundations of Health

Ginkgo, Elixir of Youth

Handbook for Herbal Healing

Medicinal Mushrooms

Milk Thistle, The Liver Herb

Natural Liver Therapy

Valerian, The Relaxing Herb

Vitex, The Women's Herb

3rd Printing, November 1995

Robert A. Barnett, Editor
Beth Baugh, Supervising Editor

Cover design, © May 1995 D.D. Dowden
Illustrations, © May 1995 Marni Fylling
Cartoon, © May 1995 Joal Morris

Botanica Press, 10226 Empire Grade, Santa Cruz, CA 95060

Table of Contents

INTRODUCTION

What is Kombucha tea? It is purported to be a mushroom that grows on sweetened tea, an ancient tonic, a cure for ailments as diverse as baldness to lethargy to cancer, an immune-boosting elixir rich in antibiotic usnic acid and liver-detoxifying glucuronic acid.

It is hardly any of these things. Rather than being a mushroom, it is a colony of yeast and bacteria. Few of the health claims are based on science, although folk history and some existing studies do suggest potential health benefits. A thorough review of the existing scientific literature fails to find any evidence that Kombucha tea, a mildly acidic fermented beverage, contains usnic acid, a compound found in certain lichens with strong antibiotic activity, as previous writers have reported. Rather than containing glucuronic acid, a potent detoxifying compound the liver produces when we consume, for example, aspirin, Kombucha tea contains gluconic acid, a common food ingredient.

That a new food or beverage would be subject to misinformation is not surprising, however. We know so little about this ancient beverage, yet it has been used for centuries in China, the Philippines, and Russia, and more recently, in Eastern Europe and Germany. It has a reputation for promoting digestion and general well-being. It may indeed have unique antibiotic and other properties. In the cultures from which it originates, Kombucha tea has a reputation for being a health-promoting beverage.

Unless it is made carefully, however, the tea can become contaminated with molds and other potential pathogens. Kombucha is often brewed at home, with Kombucha "babies," the sponge-like cellulose matrix containing the bacteria-yeast colony that grows on sugar-sweetened black tea, being passed from friend to friend, to start new batches.

So the potential for a friendly epidemic is there. For that reason alone, its use in patients with HIV or AIDS, at least until further research clarifies the potential risks and benefits, is not recommended. Its use for diabetics is controversial (perhaps because it contains about 3-4% simple sugars). For anyone who does want to participate in the "Kombucha craze," safe preparation methods are essential. Fortunately, the rules for safe tea making are fairly simple.

Clearly we need to know more about this beverage. The health claims are extraordinary, both here in the United States, in its brief life here, and in the countries of origin. Many may turn out to be groundless, but others may turn out to be based on solid physiology.

The purpose of this book is to separate fact from fiction, provide an historical context, lay out the best available knowledge of the bacteria and yeasts that go into the fermentation process of Kombucha, and explore how these may affect health. We will discuss safety issues thoroughly and provide instructions for the safe preparation of this sweet-sour beverage. While it may not be a panacea for all the ills humans are heir to, Kombucha tea is a traditional fermented beverage used in many cultures to promote well-being. Let us explore whether and how it can fit into a healthful lifestyle.

Panacea — Or Traditional Fermented Beverage?

Suzanne is a professional woman in her late 40s who lives in New York City. She started to make Kombucha tea about a year ago, when a visiting friend from California recommended it. "My friend said it helped a friend of hers get over cancer," recalls Suzanne. "I'm a very mind-over-matter sort of person, and I thought 'This is silly.' That's how I felt when she was here."

But she tried it anyway. "I have cystic fibroid disease. I've had it for 10 years. Every few years, the doctors aspirate the cysts. It's not cancer, but it scares me. It was happening again. I don't like going to doctors. So my friend said she'd send me a mushroom. After a week of drinking the tea, the lumps went away. When I went home for Christmas, I didn't drink any tea for two weeks; they came back. That's weird. I don't know what it's all about, but it's pretty wonderful.

"To be honest, I'm not really crazy about the tea. I don't particularly like the taste. Actually, it tastes different every time. Sometimes it's sweeter, other times it's bubbly. Sometimes, when you separate a new baby from the mushroom, it hisses at you. I drink about three quarters of a juice glass, maybe 6 ounces, once a day, as soon as I get up, then I don't eat for at least 30 minutes. I'm sort of a vegetarian, but I still drink coffee and smoke cigarettes. I figure the tea won't hurt me; it seems to help me, and maybe it will counteract some of my bad habits.

"You know, the health chain letter that my friend sent me made all sorts of promises. These haven't come true. My hair is still getting gray. It doesn't help the skin problems I sometimes have. I'm not any thinner. I'm still getting wrinkles. That's part of aging. I can't help it. I take Kombucha for this one specific thing, and it seems to help."

Testimonials for Kombucha abound. Suzanne's is actually one of the more cautious ones. Consider this list, which was sent over a bulletin board on Compuserve recently. "It prevents certain types of cancer; in Manchuria, where it originally comes from, there hasn't been detected a single case of cancer," the bulletin board posting begins. It goes on to add that AIDS patients go into remission, that it "eliminates wrinkles and helps the removal of brown liver spots on hands," that it "reduces hot-flash discomforts during menopause." Kombucha, the author continues, also "helps constipation, helps muscular aches and pains in the shoulders and neck," "helps bronchitis, asthma, and coughs," "helps with allergies," "helps kidney problems," "has proven useful in cataracts and other formations on the cornea," and "helps heal diseases." The same missive also claims that the Kombucha tea lowers cholesterol ("softens veins and arteries"), helps cuts heal faster, cleanses the gall bladder, helps colitis and "nervous" stomachs, helps migraine headaches, helps arthritis and gout, stops infectious diarrhea, helps the burning of fat ("and therefore helps to lose weight"), helps insomnia, gives increased energy and less need of sleep, helps the liver work more efficiently, and helps to level off glucose and "sudden drops of blood sugar in diabetics." Finally, the author writes, this wondrous tea "helps digestion, helps get rid of adult acne, and helps multiple sclerosis." Other enthusiasts claim Kombucha retards aging and cures irritability, mental fatigue, and low sex drive. To my knowledge, no studies exist to support such claims.

Some Kombucha believers are more focused about their expectations, if not less enthusiastic. Stan Russell, 70, is a psychiatrist in

Mill Valley, in Marin County, just north of San Francisco. He's been drinking the tea for over a year." At the time I started to drink it, I had painful arthritis in both my knees. I don't have that anymore. I also used to get tired in the afternoon, but I don't anymore."

He drinks about four ounces a day. When he makes it, using black tea and white sugar, he often adds a little white vinegar, to help get the fermentation process started, and to protect the brew against contamination.

"Now I brew lots of it, as much as 14 gallons at a time. I pass it out to my friends. I have a friend who suffers from the effects of breast implants, and this relieves her discomforts." He says he's seen it help one friend with colon cancer, another with multiple sclerosis. "She's had MS for 26 years, and since she started drinking the tea about a year ago, she's had steady improvement, in her eyesight, her hearing, her mind. Now she can speak distinctly and articulately."

From a scientific standpoint, such testimonials, or anecdotal evidence, are not enough to establish a true benefit. Human beings have powerful innate healing abilities, and the power of belief is a strong healing "agent" indeed. Simply believing that something will help you often does, especially in complex diseases that involve both the body and the mind. Unfortunately, there has been very little true scientific study of Kombucha, certainly not in this country, where it is only about 15 years old, nor even in Europe or Asia.

There is, however, a rich cultural context. Where it is known best, Kombucha is rarely considered a cure-all. "In China, a lot of people brew it at home, and use it as a tonic—like ginseng," explains Devin Fann of Ontario, Canada. His father, Kuni Fann, Ph.D., a professor of philosophy, brought the "tea fungus" from China about 10 years ago. He started to brew it and combine it with several herbs and flowers, including hibiscus, rosehips, hawthorn berries, honeysuckle, chrysanthemum, spearmint, lemon grass, chamomile, licorice root, and Siberian ginseng, and eventually, market it under the name "Yin-Yang Harmony Drink." Says Devin Fann, "The Kombucha we make is pasteurized. It doesn't have live bacterial cultures. But it's not like yogurt—it's not the bacteria that are beneficial. It's the acids themselves that have antibacterial and antioxidant properties. Like vinegar.

"Kombucha is a healthy alternative to soft drinks. It's not medicine by any stretch of the imagination. As far as we know, it's a preventive, good for your immune system. It started in

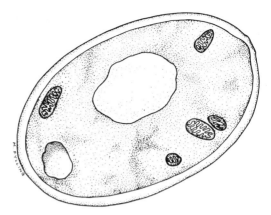

A typical yeast cell.

China, then moved to Russia and Europe, where it's been used as a tonic for a long time."

As a traditional food and beverage that has such widespread use over hundreds of years, Kombucha tea probably has some health benefits, but the fantastic claims that are made for it are undoubtedly overblown. I consider Kombucha tea simply a healthful (when made properly) and to some, a flavorful beverage that is fun to make at home. The social aspect of discussing how our Kombucha is doing, how well it grows on different teas, and sharing the "offspring" with friends and even strangers, is an important part of its allure.

Anatomy of "The Tea Beast"

Kombucha tea is a fermented beverage, usually home-brewed. How it is made is one of its fascinations. The Kombucha mother—also called "The Tea Beast," or Kambotscha, "tea mushroom" or Fungus Japonicus, and mother of vinegar or "vinegar plant"—is a tough jelly-like "skin." In Japan it is also called "Manchurian Tea," as well as "Kouchakinoko," which means, literally, black tea (Koucha) mushroom (Kinoko).

In actuality the Kombucha mother is not a mushroom at all, but a complex association or symbiosis of yeasts (which are simple fungi) and bacteria embedded in a pure cellulose "pancake." The identity of these organisms is known, but the exact microbial composition depends upon the specific culture. When the Kombucha skin is grown on a blend of black tea and sugar, it has the power to transform the resulting liquid into a refreshingly sweet and sour, lightly sparkling beverage with a fruity fragrance, reminiscent of apple cider, which is enjoyed throughout Asia and Europe. The liquid is also called "tea kvass" or "tea cider." In this book, we will refer to the skin as the "Kombucha mother," and the liquid as "Kombucha tea."

When the Kombucha skin or mother is cultured on an infusion of tea (which provides nitrogen, vitamins and minerals, and other essential nutritive substances) and sugar, its yeasts flourish, transforming the sugar into small amounts of alcohol. Most of that alcohol is ultimately changed to acetic acid, up to 3%, by the bacteria, which also thrive on B vitamins produced by the yeast. This process gives the "tea" a sweet and sour smell of fermenting apple cider. The finished tea is reported to contain on average between 0.5 and 1% alcohol, as well as lesser amounts of lactic acid, tartaric acid, malic acid, malonic acid, citric acid, and oxalic acid (List & Hammer, 1973). When black tea is used to make the nutrient solution upon which the organism grows, small amounts of caffeine are present, depending on the brewing method and the caffeine content of the original tea. During the fermentation process, the

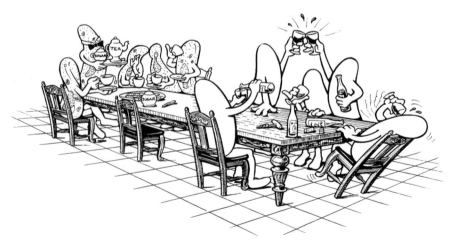

The yeasts enjoy some tea with their sugar while the bacteria go a little overboard with the alcohol!

caffeine is not entirely degraded and is still present in the finished tea (Hermann, 1927). Simple sugar content in the finished product, even when table sucrose is used, is minimal, about 3-5%. (We provide a nutritional analysis of a typical batch later in this book).

Making Kombucha tea is related to the vinegar-making process. Vinegar itself has long had a reputation for promoting well-being (Bragg and Bragg, n.d.). Kombucha tea is actually a mild vinegar. German authors Steiger & Steinegger (1957) commented on this similarity: "It can be assumed that the same fungus was used in the Volga area to make Teekwaas (Kombucha) one time and vinegar another time. Thus, it can be said that tea fungus and vinegar fungus are formed in the same manner by a community of bacteria and yeasts. It is important in the use of both fungi that the vinegar is made directly from sugar and not, as in industrial production, from alcoholic liquids. This is probably only possible because of the fermenting yeasts; vinegar bacteria alone would hardly be able to transform sugar into acetic acid to such an extent."

Over the last 50 years, and probably much longer, Kombucha tea has enjoyed cycles of popularity in many European countries, throughout Asia and the U.S., and is currently experiencing a re-awakening of interest, with numerous reports in the popular press. Kombucha tea can be considered a traditional fermented food; in the Philippines, as we'll see, the Kombucha mother is eaten as dessert, a delicacy called "nata." Its origins are probably in China.

Origins —
And Worldwide Diffusion

The infusion of Kombucha is said to have been extremely popular as a folk remedy for thousands of years (Fasching, 1994). The first recorded use of the tea was during the Chinese empire of the Qin-Dynasty in 221 B.C. (Frank, 1991). It was known as "The Remedy for Immortality" or "The Divine Tsche". The "Tsche" (meaning tea) was said to be introduced in Japan by the Korean doctor Kombu in 414 B.C. (Fasching, 1994). One German article, however, argues that the origins may have been in Russia (Steiger & Steinegger, 1957).

Frank (1991) offers an explanation of the name, Kombucha. He writes that the name originated from the Japanese name for a sea-weed, kombu, and from the word "cha," meaning tea. His contention is that someone may have made the culture from kombu tea, and the name was erroneously transferred to the culture. Kombu tea is still sold throughout Japan and is very popular. Kombu seaweed tea is available in powdered form and is widely available in stores, tea shops, and other establishments.

About 20 years ago, the "Manchurian mushroom" experienced a resurgence of popularity in Japan. Tomoko Nakamura, now an American businesswoman whose mother forced her to drink it when she was in a Tokyo high school, relates that all of her mother's friends were growing it then. "It was in every apartment and house, and it was all the rage for a year or two, after which time its use died out." Tomoko was stopped from using the tea by the family doctor who said he didn't know anything about it and was concerned. Last year, another revival in Kombucha brewing started and continues today.

After its first introduction in Japan more than 2,000 years ago, Kombucha tea came to be used in the Philippines, Java, India, Russia, and Eastern European countries. For instance, C.H. Gadd from the Tea Research Institute of Ceylon, in a 1933 speech before English tea growers and their families, said that the drink was very popular in Java because the indigenous people have an aversion to alcoholic drinks (Gadd, 1933).

In the Philippines, a kind of Kombucha is popular as a desert delicacy. Instead of the usual black tea and sugar, the mother is grown on fruit juice and sugar, especially coconut milk, and the bacterium that produces the mother in Kombucha (*Acetobacter aceti sbsp. xylinum*) has been identified from Nata cultures. Researchers from the National Institute of Science and Technology in Manila found that the Nata "organism" is the same as the mother of vinegar (Lapuz et al, 1967). The cellulose pancake is sold in the sweet and sour coconut and sugar liquid in the markets under names such as nata de piña (pineapple Nata), or nata de coco (coconut Nata), and other names, depending on the fruit that is added to the original culture. The pancake is cut into cubes, cooked, and eaten along with the liquid.

The same researchers report that the production of Nata is practiced in homes, and a commercial industry is growing because of the abundant amount of coconut water that is available as a by-product of the production of copra from coconuts, which are widely grown on the island. A later report from the same institute in Manila emphasized that Nata production was increasing, and due to its popularity, was being introduced into foreign markets (Gallardo-de Jesus et al, 1971). Consumers are reported to have specific preferences for Nata that is either soft, medium, or firm-textured, and the researchers studied the production of Nata with varying starting fruits to determine what resulting texture each would produce. A soft pancake was produced when tomato and sugar were used as a starting material, a medium texture from pineapple, orange, guava, apple, radish, and mulberry fruits, and a firm-textured product was only produced from saba fruit, which is not generally available outside of Asia. The color of the Nata pancake varied from creamy white to yellow to pinkish.

Kombucha was reportedly introduced into Germany from Russia by sailors about 1911 (Gadd, 1933). It is said that Kombucha enjoyed wide popularity until World War II when black tea and sugar (with which it is grown) became scarce (Fasching, 1994).

Modern Use — And Modern Claims

The first scientific publication in the German literature is dated 1913 (Steiger & Steinegger, 1957). A Baltic report is dated 1915. A publication from 1914 documented the use of the tea in various regions of Russia: St. Petersburg, Wilna, Witebsk, Kursk, Odessa, and the Caucasus. In 1915, according to one report, a Polish pharmacist prepared a mild but effective laxative based on a "Russian folk remedy," the so-called "miracle fungus," "Volga fungus," or Teekwass fungus." By 1925, Kombucha appears to have found its way to common German use. It was also used in Denmark. In an overview of the drugs for the year 1927 Hahmann (1929) calls the fungus "Indian" and "Japanese tea fungus," "Russian jelly-fish," "Volga jelly-fish," and "Kombucha;" several years prior the fungus is said to have appeared in Hamburg for the first time; interest in it is said to have been enormous and supposedly increased in 1928. That year, the tea was already an advertised commodity. Even then, concerned medical authorities warned against exaggerated reports of "alleged successful treatments of a suspiciously large number of different kinds of illnesses," write Steiger and Steinegger (1957). They reported that after World War II, use of Kombucha apparently spread to Italy, France, and Spain. Reiss (1994) reports that Kombucha tea has long been considered a refreshing drink with mild laxative effects because of the simple hydroxy acids (lactic, gluconic, etc.). Historically, he says that it was originally introduced into Germany by Russian and German prisoners of war.

During the 1960s the Waischenfelder Apotheke was recommending Kombucha to be taken daily as a preventative and therapeutic remedy for such diverse ailments as the onset of arteriosclerosis, constipation, physical and mental fatigue, low sex drive, and convalescence. According to Fasching (1994), Hans Irion, who was then director of the Brunswick Pharmaceutical Academy, also advocated its use for high blood pressure, nervousness, overweight, sports activities, excessive mental activity, and symptoms of aging. Fasching also claims to have observed a reduction in colds by some people taking the tea as a preventive remedy. Also, because of its reputed purifying effects, it is reported to be a good protectant against the daily assault on our bodies from various environmental pollution. Some use Kombucha once a year as one would take a spring tonic. *Hagers Handbuch* (List & Hörhammer, 1973) states that "Combucha" is used as a folk remedy for edema, arteriosclerosis, gout, constipation, and stones. To my knowledge, there is no scientific data to back up any of these claims.

In the 1960s a German doctor named Sklenar developed a "biological cancer therapy" using mainly Kombucha, which he had learned about in Russia during the war. He had unusual views about cancer, considering it to be a viral-based disease, which could be diagnosed by looking into the irises of the eye. Sklenar theorized that the glucuronic acid, reported to be in Kombucha, causes detoxification, based on its known detoxifying function in the liver. The glucuronic acid forms conjugates with metabolic waste products and harmful substances, such as drugs or poisons, thereby facilitating the detoxification process (Fasching, 1994).

regard to Kombucha's effect on metabolism, particularly concerning its "detoxifying function" through its linkage with D-glucuronate (R. Fasching, 1988; K. H., 1986; H. Korner, 1987; U. Ruckert, 1987).

More credible tests are needed to substantiate this theory, however. One laboratory analysis which was commissioned by a leading manufacturer and distributor of a commercial kombucha tea product has found about 0.4% of glucuronic acid. However, it does contain gluconic acid, a common acid formed from glucose. Nor are there clinical trials to support the effectiveness of Kombucha in cases of cancer, although it is being promoted as an "effective biological cancer therapy." Sklenar reports a few anecdotal cases but did not do any credible studies. The Swiss Society for Oncology and the Swiss Cancer Association, after careful studies of the available literature, as well as other obtainable information, have not found data that would support Kombucha's use in the treatment of cancer (Hauser, 1990). After my own thorough search, I must come to the same conclusion, though further studies and experience may prove me wrong.

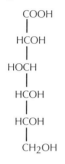

Gluconic acid

Acetic acid and lactic acid, however, may have mild detoxifying effects; they have been widely reported in the literature on fermented foods to retard the growth of harmful bacteria while promoting the growth of beneficial bacteria in the intestine. As such, it may be placed in the context of traditional fermented foods, such as sauerkraut and yogurt.

As previously mentioned, numerous health claims have been made in the popular literature, as well as by businesses who are selling the culture. Today, those claims include helping AIDS patients to boost their T cell count. There does not appear to be any data to support this, either, other than anecdotal. Indeed, some Kombucha critics argue that it is a particularly dangerous beverage for people with compromised immunity to experiment with. "People with AIDS are not even supposed to drink tap water," says mushroom grower Paul Stamets, a prominent critic of the Kombucha craze. He reports that in two cases, HIV-positive patients, who were

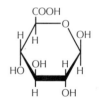

Glucuronic acid

asymptomatic before drinking Kombucha, wound up "with full-blown AIDS." Such anecdotes are themselves not scientific, of course. AIDS watchdog groups have also called for extreme caution, however. Says natural medicine advocate Andrew Weil, MD, "I have heard stories of HIV-positive persons becoming very sick after drinking it. It is potentially dangerous."

One claim for Kombucha tea that is certainly not surprising is that of weight loss. Not surprising because obesity is prevalent and rising in the United States, and, after all, any good panacea worth its salt should be able to produce substantial weight-loss in its users. During my close association with the herb and supplement industry, I have seen a number of weight-loss formulas make substantial amounts of money for their manufacturers.

Although Kombucha tea has no studies showing that it is effective for this use, at least one study performed in Nigeria lends a little preliminary support (Kwanashie et al, 1989). In two different experiments, researchers fed mice a popular fermented tea from 15 to 100% of their diet and noted a reduction in food intake and a reversible weight-loss in the animals. The tea is called Kargasok tea, which the researchers claim is similar to Kombucha tea. Though it is not certain that the microbial content is the same, the tea is brewed on black tea and sugar and is said to have a "pleasant wine taste." The authors speculate that alcohol itself might be responsible for at least some of the tea's activity. It is also known that Kombucha tea contains caffeine, a known stimulant, which might further explain the appetite reduction. Unfortunately, there are too many unknowns about this study, since there was no analysis of alcohol or caffeine reported by the authors. The tea could have had even higher concentrations of these substances than Kombucha tea, which is known to contain about as much caffeine as 1/20 a cup of coffee in a daily dose of 4 ounces three times a day, and from 0.5 to 1.0% alcohol, which would amount to 1/4 to 1/2 of a weak (2% ethanol) beer sipped over an entire day. This would hardly be enough for any major appetite suppression to occur.

We have already stated that Kombucha tea contains neither usnic acid nor glucuronic acid, both of which are proffered to explain purported health benefits. Because much of the scientific analysis of the beverage is decades old, many of the organisms that are still cited in contemporary writings are actually outdated names. The current names of these yeasts and bacteria provide some insight into what Kombucha tea truly is, and how it may exert whatever health benefits it does actually confer.

Let us look a little closer inside this sweet-sour, fermented, acidic, slightly carbonated beverage. Whether you are drinking the tea now or are considering adding it to your health regimen, the question remains: What is in Kombucha?

The Microbiology of Kombucha Tea

Kombucha is not any single organism or "mushroom," as is sometimes reported. Rather it is a "community" of yeasts and bacteria living in a thick pellicle, or rubbery skin. Far from being dangerous because of the presence of these organisms, this kind of association is an extremely common and beneficial one.

Many traditional fermented foods, which are mainstays of indigenous diets, such as kefir from the Caucasus, leben from Egypt, and kumiss from Russia and Asia, are made with the help of specific communities of these organisms. These foods are as much a part of many traditional cultures as the language itself—and have probably been known and used for hundreds, if not thousands, of years.

The bacteria and yeasts in the Kombucha "mother of vinegar" interact in complex and mysterious ways, first one active and pre-dominant, depending on varying conditions of temperature, pH, and sugar concentration. Then, the other rises to dominance.

First, when a mixture of black tea and sugar (or any other appropriate substrate) is brewed, and a Kombucha mother of vinegar is added to it, yeasts feed on the sugar, minerals and vitamins, and other nutrients in the solution. They multiply rapidly, producing alcohol. The environment created by the yeasts, rich in B vitamins, then allows the bacteria to go to work, converting the alcohol into acetic acid. *Voilá*, vinegar is created. *Acetobacter aceti* subsp. *xylinum* is known to form a tough skin or pellicle on top of batches of brewing vinegar, traditionally known as a "mother of vinegar."

This bacterium has also been identified from Kombucha, along with other organisms associated with the production of vinegar.

As the bacteria multiply, the number of yeast cells declines. Many yeasts, however, have an ability to attach to surfaces, such as the cellulose matrix produced by the Kombucha bacteria *A. aceti* subsp. *xylinum.* The yeasts may form small colonies in this cellulose mat. When a Kombucha "baby" is placed into a new batch of tea and sugar, the yeasts go to work again.

Thus, a cyclic balance forms between the bacteria and the yeast. It is a miraculous dance of life and biochemistry, which works its magic on complex and simple food molecules alike, producing vitamins, sterols, ethanol, simple acids, such as acetic acid, and other metabolites.

Scientists have speculated why bacteria produce cellulose, especially one as thick and solid as the Kombucha mother. The most accepted theories have to do with the bacteria's ability to compete and thrive on their usual natural substrates where they naturally occur, for instance rotting fruit. Williams and Cannon (1989) from the Department of Biology, University of North Carolina studied *A. aceti* subsp. *xylinum* and the cellulose "pellicle" (i.e. Kombucha mother) it produces, which they say is composed of bundles of cellulose microfibrils created by an enzyme they produce, *cellulose synthetase.* They argue that the cellulose matrix may help keep them close to the air, which contains oxygen, which they need for optimum growth. It may also enhance the ability of the bacteria to multiply in large masses of cells or colonies, increasing their ability

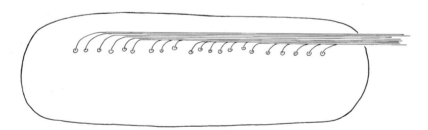

Acetobacter aceti subsp. **xylinum** produces pure cellulose strands from pores in its cell wall. These fibers can be used to make clothes, paper and other products now made from trees — the creator of the Kombucha mother may be a friend to our planetary environment.

to compete with other organisms vying for the same food. Finally, the opaque quality of the cellulose may help protect the bacteria from damage by ultraviolet light. (Cellulose is a unique polymer compound produced in nature. It gives plant cell walls structure and form, and may in the future turn out to be an inexpensive, low-pollution source of paper, artificial leather, and other products. Cellulose fibers are insoluble in most liquid solvents, and rigid, and although extremely light, have been said to have a tensile strength which compares with steel).

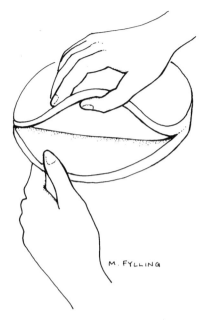

M. FYLLING

The Kombucha mother eventually separates into layers — pass one on to a friend, perhaps have it for dinner, but don't flush it — it can continue growing and clog your drain!

The Kombucha "mother" is very closely related to this mother of vinegar. Well, more than "closely related." In fact, they are one and the same! In traditional vinegar making, a thick cellulose mat is formed. This is what we now call the Kombucha mother, or, when it separates, the Kombucha baby.

So a conversation about Kombucha is really a conversation about vinegar. Vinegar is an ancient fermented food that is said to have a number of health benefits, which we will explore below.

Kombucha Organisms

In 1928, Hermann reported on his identification in Kombucha of two bacteria, *Bacterium xylinum* Brown and *B. xylinoides* Henneberg. Both are now known to be the same organism: *Acetobacter aceti* subsp. *xylinum* (Brown) *comb. nov*. He also reported a second bacterium, *B. gluconicum* Hermann, now known as

Gluconobacter oxydans subsp. *suboxydans comb. nov.*; it is named after its ability to form gluconic acid.

Researchers have subsequently determined that Kombucha is a symbiotic association of "vinegar bacteria," mainly *A. aceti* subsp. *xylinum*, which produces the pure cellulose mat or "pellicle" that we associate with the name "Kombucha." It also contains *Acetobacter ketogenum* (sic) (Walker and Thomas), now known as *Acetobacter aceti* [Pasteur] Beijerinck).

Nest-like masses of yeast cells are embedded in this cellulose mat. These include: *Pichia fermentans* Lodder, *Saccharomyces apiculatus* Reess, which is now called *Kloeckera apiculata* (Reess Emend. Klöcker) Janke (1928). *Saccharomycodes ludwigii* Hansen, and *Schizosaccharomyces pombe* Lindner (List & Hörhammer, 1973; *Bergey's Manual of Determinative* Bacteriology, 9th ed., 1994). It is entirely possible that other bacteria and yeasts are present in a given batch of Kombucha tea, depending on the type of tea used, the temperature, the starting culture, the percentage and type of sugar used, and other factors.

There is no evidence that the tea or the Kombucha mother contain usnic acid, a lichen acid that has antibiotic properties, nor do any chemical analyses of Kombucha tea identify glucuronic acid as a constituent or metabolic by-product. If it is present, it occurs in minor amounts. Gluconic acid, which is a major component, is chemically distinct from glucuronic acid and is not used by the liver for detoxification (Osol et al, 1955).

A number of yeasts and bacteria, all of which are commonly found in traditional fermented foods have been identified from the Kombucha community. In the following section, I identify these organisms, with the modern scientific names (Buchanan and Gibbons, 1974; Holt, 1994; Kreger-Van Rij, 1984).

The following organisms have been identified from Kombucha so far, but researchers who have studied Kombucha tea are clear that the exact species of microorganisms may vary slightly, depending on the starting culture (List and Hufschmidt, 1959). Most books and articles on Kombucha report names that are long since outdated, leading to confusion. In the following table, I give the outdated names (for reference), as well as the currently accepted names and the person's name who first identified and described the organism.

The first two bacteria I describe are called "vinegar bacteria," because they play an important role in the conversion of ethyl alcohol to acetic acid in the production of vinegar.

Kombucha Bacteria

Acetobacter ketogenum (sic) (Walker and Thomas in Bousfield, Wright and Walker 1947) is now *Acetobacter aceti* (Pasteur) (Beijerinck 1898).

Description: prefer alcohol-rich environments, as opposed to *Gluconobacter* spp. which likes a sugar-rich environment; "aceti" means "vinegar." Members of the genus *Acetobacter* have a requirement for an environment rich in B-vitamins, which can be supplied by yeasts. The association of yeasts and bacteria in Kombucha may be a symbiosis, whereby each species contributes to the milieu in which they all live in order to create an environment where all can flourish. *A. aceti* will grow in a solution that is high in simple sugars, primarily glucose, and can utilize ethyl alcohol as an additional source of energy only when acetic acid is also present. *Gluconobacter oxydans* subsp. *suboxydans* can produce acetic acid from ethyl alcohol, thus supporting the growth of *A. aceti*.

Bacterium xylinoides (Henneberg) (Shimwell 1948) is now *Acetobacter aceti* subsp. *xylinum* (Brown) *comb. nov.*

Description: ellipsoidal to rod-shaped straight or slightly curved cells; oxidizes ethanol to acetic acid; acetate and lactate are oxidized to CO_2 and water (overoxidizers); grows readily on ethanol; surface growth forms a tough, leathery pellicle, composed of cellulose; the main organism that is responsible for the thick, rubbery "film" in Kombucha, which is technically called a zooglea.

Bacterium gluconicum (Hermann, 1928) is now Gluconobacter oxydans subsp. suboxydans (Kluyver and de Leeuw) comb. nov.

Description: the cells are ellipsoidal to rod-shaped and often have 3-8 polar flagella; oxidizes ethanol to acetic acid; optimum temperature range, 25-30 deg. C. Occurrence: souring fruits, vegetables, beer, apple cider, wine, baker's yeast, garden soil, South African "kaffir beer."

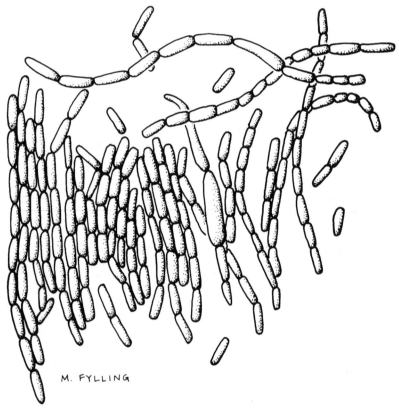

M. FYLLING

A colony of *Acetobacter aceti* subsp. *xylinum,* the most important of the vinegar bacteria in kombucha tea and the creator of the pure cellulose Kombucha mother.

Kombucha Yeasts and Yeast-Like Organisms

Besides bacteria, a number of yeasts have been identified from Kombucha. A yeast is a simple one-celled organism that is a unicellular fungus which reproduces by budding or fission (vegetative reproduction) or by the production of minute germ-cells called spores (sexual reproduction). Budding is the process by which a yeast cell develops other similar cells as a branch, sometimes bilaterally from the "mother cell." The end adjacent to the "mother" cell then constricts, releasing the "daughter cell." Fission is the formation of daughter cells by cross-wall formation and subsequent splitting and separation.

Many yeasts are beneficial organisms which have been "cultivated" by humans for many centuries to help produce beverages and foods. For instance, the oldest known sedative and sleep-promoting drug is manufactured by a yeast—ethyl alcohol. While some yeasts are known to be harmful to humans, like *Candida albicans* which is associated with life-threatening infections in people with compromised immune function, none of the yeasts identified from Kombucha have been reported to be pathogenic (disease-promoting). However, it should be noted, in people with compromised immune systems, even non-pathogenic microorganisms can multiply prodigiously, causing illness.

Like the higher fungi, some yeasts belong to the *Ascomycetes*, which produce spores in sacs, and *Basidiomycetes*, producing spores on club-like structures called basidia. A third group of yeasts, the "imperfect yeasts," are associated with both of the other two groups.

All of the yeasts that have been identified from Kombucha are in the family *Saccharomycetaceae*, which are all related to the *Ascomycetes*. Different subfamilies and genera (a group of individual species) are delineated by determining exactly how budding or fission takes place, the shape and size of the spores, and the type of chemical process the organism uses to ferment sugars, as well as what other compounds (like nitrates) it takes up, metabolizes, or produces. These taxonomic characteristics are well beyond the scope of this work, but I am giving a little background about yeasts so that the reader will have some understanding about where these fascinating organisms fit into the scheme of things.

Yeasts are extremely common in nature, living and hibernating in the soil until conditions are right for rapid growth and reproduction. Conditions which favor this are warmth, moisture, and the presence of various sugars such as glucose, sucrose, and lactose. Ripe fruits are especially favorable environments for the development of yeasts, and yeasts acting on these sugars often produce vinegar and alcoholic beverages. On the other hand, yeasts living in soil are killed rapidly by exposure to heat and the ultraviolet light in sunlight. Yeast cells can be transported by the wind, by bees (and by honey) and other insects, and by animals.

Yeasts contain a high percentage of protein, vitamins and minerals, and sterols, especially ergosterol, which can convert to vitamin D when exposed to sunlight. Commercially, yeasts are important as the organisms mainly responsible for the transformation of sugar into alcohol (about 40-45% of glucose to ethanol) and for the production of beer, wine, and other alcoholic beverages (brewer's yeast is often cultivated strains of *Saccharomyces cerevisiae*)—it is hard to decide at times whether humans owe yeasts a debt of gratitude or should consider them a curse for this favor. From alcohol, yeasts produce acetic acid and vinegar. The rising of bread, as well as the creation of the sour flavor in "sourdough" breads, is an action brought about by the production of gases by complex mixtures of yeasts (especially "baker's yeast", strains of *Saccharomyces cerevisiae*) and bacteria.

The cocoa that is so popular worldwide, for the production of chocolate drinks and candy, is produced by a fermentation process of the ripe beans by yeasts. Some of the organisms responsible include *Kloeckera apiculata*, *Pichia fermentans*, and species of *Schizosaccharomyces*—all of which occur in Kombucha.

Other compounds commonly produced by all yeasts include glycerol, small amounts of higher alcohols, such as isoamyl, isobutyl, n-propyl alcohols, and even smaller amounts of n-butanol. Some yeasts (but not all) produce such compounds as acetic acid (the main component of vinegar), lactic acid, succinic acid, zymonic acid, ethyl acetate, saturated and unsaturated fatty acids, such as compounds that may make up part of the pellicle produced by Kombucha organisms, called sphingolipids, which are produced by some yeasts from glucose (1-2% is converted). Some yeasts also commonly produce coloring pigments such as carotenoids. Optimum temperature for maximum yeast growth is often from 25-30 deg. C., with the minimum temperature for growth about 2 deg. C., and the maximum about 37-40 deg. C.

Main Yeasts Found in Kombucha

Pichia fermentans (Lodder, 1932).

Description: forms pseudohyphae, spores are hat-shaped, forms a pellicle (thick skin); rapidly ferments glucose, also assimilates D-xylose, succinic acid, and citric acid; produces DL-lactic acid; 8% viable after freeze-drying, 4% after 9 months; can grow at pH 1.5, which is highly acidic.

Other sources: buttermilk (identified in Holland), some cheeses (from Italy), California olives, sputum, spoiled orange juice (also occurs in the fresh fruit), kefir, fermenting cocoa in Africa and Indonesia.

Saccharomyces apiculatus Reess is now *Kloeckera apiculata* (Reess Emend. Klöcker) Janke (1928).

Description: cells are lemon-shaped, apiculate, oval or elongate; forms a sediment; requires inositol and panthotenate for growth; strongly ferments glucose, assimilates cellobiose, creates 2-ketogluconate; most common member of the genus, widespread. It is interesting that in French wine-making districts, this yeast is often the second most-common organism, and in other cool climates worldwide, it may be the most common. In vineyards that have a history of many years of production, yeasts, which reside or hibernate in the soil, are transferred to the grapes (most likely by fruit flies) as they ripen. When the grapes are crushed, fermentation begins. The blend of wild strains of yeasts adds character and uniqueness to the wines of each district and vineyard.

Other sources: soil, flowers, common on ripe strawberries (can initiate spoilage), cherries, plums, grapes (one of the most common yeasts found in grape juices), fruit juice, rotting strawberries (can initiate spoilage)

Saccharomy-codes ludwigii Hansen (1904)

Description: cells are lemon-shaped or elongate, poorly developed pseudomycelium; forms a sediment and a ring; ferments glucose, sucrose, and raffinose, assimilates sucrose, cellobiose, raffinose; exposure to diffuse sunlight inhibits its growth.

Other sources: exudates of oak trees

Schizosaccharo-myces pombe Lindner (1893)

Description: cells are round, ellipse-shaped, or cylindrical; produces a sediment; ferments glucose, sucrose, maltose, raffinose (slightly); assimilates sucrose, maltose, raffinose; most common member of the genus; can attack larger sugar molecules than most yeasts (oligosaccharides).

Other sources: molasses, grape juice, brewer's yeast, cane sugar, apple, Bantu beer, palm wine; used in rum fermentation in Jamaica.

Note: This species of yeast is widely used in genetic research in medical science.

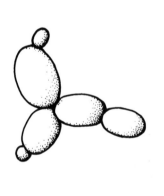 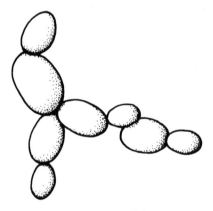

M. FYLLING

Yeasts reproduce by "budding."

Specific Constituents in Kombucha Tea: Simple Hydroxy Acids

The yeasts and bacteria create certain substances, such as acetic acid, as the Kombucha tea ferments. Some of these, such as the simple hydroxy acids (acetic, lactic, gluconic), may be responsible for part of the tea's reputed antibacterial, and other, effects. Here are the major constituents of the tea:

▶ **Acetic acid.** Kombucha tea contains between 0.4 and about 3.0% acetic acid, depending on how long it is allowed to ferment. Acetic acid is effective in killing a number of common pathogenic bacteria. For instance, in one study, two species of Salmonella were added to a salad dressing containing oil and vinegar. After 5 minutes, none of the organisms were detected after an initial inoculum of 5 x 10^6 of *S. enteritidis*. In the meat industry, acetic and lactic acid are widely used to wash animal carcasses to reduce microbacterial contamination. When acetic acid is sprayed on beef slices, for example, there are significant reductions in the potentially pathogenic bacteria *Listeria monocytogenes*, *Salmonella typhimurium*, and *E. coli*, even when the acetic acid concentration is as low as 0.5% to 2.0% (Jay, 1992).

▶ **Gluconic acid.** Kombucha tea contains about 2% of this weak acid. Our body produces large amounts of gluconic acid as a metabolic by-product of glucose. It is used in the food industry as a food preservative.

▶ **Lactic acid.** Less than 1% usually occurs in Kombucha tea, although a starting concentration of 50 g of sucrose/liter produced the highest amount. The highest concentration is usually realized after about 6-11 days at room temperature (70 degrees).

▶ **Other simple hydroxy acids.** Researchers have identified a number of other hydroxy acids from Kombucha tea in minor amounts, the composition of which is dependent on the strains of bacteria present, the temperature, and other factors. These include citric acid, tartaric acid, succinic acid, malonic acid, and oxalic acid.

Other Constituents: Caffeine, Alcohol, Sugar

A cup of Kombucha tea (5 oz) contains up to 5 mg of caffeine. A strong cup of coffee contains about 100 mg of caffeine. So it is not a significant source of caffeine.

Kombucha tea can contain ethyl alcohol in a range of from 0.4 to 1.5%, but rarely over 1%. This is a very small amount. Many beverages, even apple juice, contain minute amounts of alcohol. By law, a beverage can contain up to 0.5% alcohol and still be labeled "non-alcoholic." Sucrose (table sugar) produces the highest concentrations of alcohol in the finished tea, with 50 grams/liter of tea the optimum amount. The most effective concentration of fructose is 150 grams/liter, which produced the highest concentration of alcohol recorded by a German research group at the Microbiological Laboratory in Bad Kreuznach (Reiss, 1994). The final concentration of alcohol is also dependent on the exact ratios of the microorganisms in the symbiotic association, as well as the

Kombucha, also known as...

Combucha
Fungus Japonicus
Gout Jelly-fish
Hongo
Indian "Tea Mould"
Indian Tea Fungus
Indian Tea Mushroom
Japanese Tea Fungus
Kambotscha
Kouchakinoko
Manchu Fungus
Manchurian Fungus
Manchurian Mushroom
Miracle Fungus
Mo-Gu
Mother of Vinegar

Mushroom of Charity
Russian Jelly-fish
Tea Mushroom
Teekwass Fungus
Teepilz
The Divine Tsche
The Remedy for Immortality
The Tea Beast
Volga Fungus
Volga Jelly-fish

Kombucha Tea is also called...

Manchurian Tea
Russian Tea-vinegar
Tea beer
Tea Cider
Tea Kvass

temperature and the time the tea is allowed to ferment. The alcohol content increases over the first 6-16 days, depending on the exact microbial content of the individual cultures, and then begins to decline, as the alcohol is converted to acetic acid. Much of the sugar that is added to Kombucha at the beginning of the fermentation process is digested by the yeasts and bacteria, so the amount of sugar in the final product is fairly small. Simple sugars occur in Kombucha tea at about 4-6%, mostly glucose, sucrose, and fructose, depending on the type of sugar (honey, table sugar) that is used for the starting culture.

The tea also contains some enzymes, including amylase, invertase, and unidentified proteolytic enzymes. Yeasts contain varying amounts of enzymes that can break down large food molecules into smaller ones, increasing the efficiency of their absorption and utilization by the body. Specifically, invertase, which hydrolyzes sucrose to glucose and fructose, and lactase, which hydrolyzes lactose (milk sugar) to glucose and galactose. As is widely known, many people have lactase deficiencies and develop symptoms of diarrhea, gas, and bloating after consuming dairy products, including some specific population groups (for instance, people of African and Asian origin). Although Kombucha tea may make a contribution to the body's ability to digest lactose-containing foods, to my knowledge, this has not specifically been studied (Reed & Peppler, 1973).

A number of individual amino acids have been identified from Kombucha tea, namely lysine, alanine, tyrosine, valine, phenylalanine, leucine and esoleucine, aspartic acid, glutamic acid, serine, and threonine (List and Hufschmidt, 1959). Like the simple hydroxy acids, amino acids may contribute some health promoting aspects to the tea. After studying rice vinegar for over 30 years, a Japanese researcher (Togo, 1977) has concluded that many of vinegar's traditional health-promoting effects are dependent on the amino acid content. Similar amino acids occur in Kombucha tea as well, along with acetic acid.

Besides the major constituents listed above, Kombucha tea undoubtedly has many of the volatile compounds, such as diacetyl, acetoin, isobutyraldehyde, vanillic acid, anisaldehyde, valeraldehyde, methylisobutyl ketone, and esters of methyl, ethyl, isobutyl and isoaml alcohols, that give it its characteristic fruity, sour, and sweet smell and taste, found in traditionally-brewed alcoholic drinks and vinegars, and in Kombucha tea (Ayres et al, 1980; Gálvez, et al, 1994). To date, hundreds have been isolated and identified. The literature on these constituents is quite large and will not be reviewed here. Besides these, vitamins and minerals are also present in varying amounts.

In a 1993 article, two researchers from the University of Stuttgart-Hoheneheim, T. Kappel and R.H. Anken, analyzed the tea and found 1% ethyl acetate, 3% acetic acid, lactic and tartaric acids, amino acids, and biogenic amines (such as choline).

It is interesting to consider what differences in fermentation are created from fruit juices (like apple or grape juice) compared to a solution of black tea and sugar. One major difference in starting constituents from black tea to fruit juice is the high tannin content of black tea. Tannins are large complex molecules technically called polyphenols, that have an astringent, or drying and condensing effect, on mucous membranes in the body. They also have antibacterial effects in many cases. It has been reported that tannins can inhibit the fermentation process, which leads to a higher finished sugar content and lower alcohol content. This may be a factor in Kombucha's relatively low maximum alcohol content, which seems to be about 0.5-1.5%, and the relatively high simple sugar content of 3-4%. Until more is known about the safety of making Kombucha from substrates other than black tea and white sugar, however, experimentation with other liquids as a fermentation base should be done cautiously. Vinegar itself is made from many substrates, such as apple juice, honey, and other fruits.

Other constituents that are known to be produced during the alcohol fermentation process that are likely to be found in Kombucha include glycerin, the higher alcohols, acetaldehyde, further aldehydes and ketones, volatile acids, and esters. The compounds undoubtedly contribute to the overall taste and aroma of Kombucha, and they are commonly found in wines and vinegars.

Laboratory Analysis of Kombucha Tea

We collected a sample of Kombucha tea, in a sterile container, from a household that had no previous knowledge of our request, and sent it directly to a certified food lab (Irvine Analytical Laboratories, Inc.) for analysis. The tea was made with 5 bags of black tea to 3 quarts of water, and one cup of table sugar and had been fermenting for exactly 1 week. We received the following results.

▶ **Simple Acids**

Gluconic acid	1.9%
Acetic acid	0.5%
Lactic acid	0.7%

▶ **Microbiological**

Yeast	5.1×10^4 CFU/mL
Mold	<10 CFU mL
Total Plate Count	363 CFU/mL

▶ **Pathogen screen**

E. coli	Negative
Coliforms	Negative
Salmonella	Negative
Staphylococcus aureus	Negative

▶ **Sugars**

Fructose	0.68%
Glucose	3.25%
Sucrose	0.27%
Maltose	None Detected
Lactose	None Detected

▶ **Other Constituents**

Caffeine	3.42 mg/100 ml

This is more or less in line with the scientific literature. Gluconic acid is expected in large amounts; it is produced by *Gluconobacter oxydans* subsp. *suboxydans comb. nov.* Acetic acid is 0.5%, which is lower than I expected; up to 4% is reported in vinegar. It is certain that the longer the Kombucha tea is left to brew, the more acetic acid is produced. Most normal batches will probably contain somewhere between 0.5 and 3%, which can be roughly estimated by taste—the more sour and vinegary, the more acetic acid is present. The quantity of lactic acid is low, and this amount is expected, based on other literature.

The amount of caffeine is fairly low, but may be higher in other batches, depending on how many tea bags are used in the original black tea, whether green tea is used (should impart less caffeine to the Kombucha tea), and the brewing method (temperature and length of time the tea is steeped). The total sugar content was about 4.2%—that is about 4 grams in a 3 1/2 ounce cup of tea, or about a teaspoon. The total sugar in this batch was made up of fructose, glucose, and sucrose.

The high yeast count is also expected, and this means that the tea is relatively early in its brewing cycle. Later in the fermentation process, the yeasts decline, the acetic acid-bacteria count rises (it was low at the time of testing), and the acetic acid content of the tea goes up. Yeasts, besides providing enzymes, also produce various B vitamins, so it is likely that this tea is a good source of B vitamins and provides some protein as well. The level of usable protein in food yeast is probably between 20 and 30%, though some methods of estimation put it at up to 45%. The limiting amino acid is methionine, but lysine is high. Kombucha tea is probably a fair supplemental source of B vitamins, even B12, which is often lacking in the diet of people who eat mostly vegetable foods. It is a poor source of protein, although not necessarily insignificant. Reed and Peppler (1973) in their book *Yeast Technology*, conclude in their chapter on "Feed and Food Yeasts," that "The contribution of yeast to protein nutrition and vitamin nutrition is undoubtedly worthwhile."

The mold count was extremely low, which is positive, and the *E. coli*, coliforms, salmonella, and *Staph. aureus* were not found at all in the tea, which is very good. When made according to standard instructions, with clean hands and utensils, Kombucha tea can be very safe. We will return to this issue in the safety section and again in the section that gives instructions for making the tea.

The Benefits of
Traditional Fermented Foods

Kombucha tea is a traditional fermented food, and its health effects are perhaps best understood in that context. "Cultured" foods are foods that have some kind of bacteria, fungus, or other organism growing on or in them which enhance the food's flavor, digestibility, or nutritional value, as well as acting as a preservative. Examples of cultured foods (and drinks) traditionally eaten in Europe, the Mediterranean area, and/or the Middle East include yogurt, sauerkraut, kefir, olives, pickles, and of course beer, wine, vinegar, cheese, cottage cheese, and buttermilk. Cultured foods traditionally eaten in certain parts of Asia include various soy sauces, shoyu or tamari, tempeh, mochi, amasake, and kimchee, as well as beers and wines.

It is difficult to say how far back in history people first made use of cultured foods. Soured milk is frequently mentioned in the Bible, and "soured milk of kine and goat's milk" mixed with fat were mentioned by Moses as one of the foods given to his people by Jehovah. Leben raib, made from fermented goat, cow, or buffalo milk, was mentioned as an important food item in the Middle East since antiquity. Of course these are only references from Judeo-Christian history. Fermented foods were also important in many other ancient cultures as well.

Although it is not certain when and where cultured foods were discovered, it is clear why they became popular. Aside from having enhanced flavor and digestibility, cultured foods have another quality that was valuable in ancient times: natural resistance to putrefaction, or spoiling. Today many people use artificial (and not especially healthful) preservatives and refrigeration to protect food from spoilage. But before the advent of these methods, culturing or fermentation was a simple, yet effective, way to preserve foods.

There are really two general ways to preserve foods by natural processes. One is to put a substance on a food to prevent putrefaction. For instance, people discovered in ancient times that vinegar, lemon juice, and lactic acid from sour milk, could preserve foods for some time.

The second method, however, is the one we are interested in here. This is to rely on fermentation of the food itself to produce substances that will preserve it. This is what a cultured food is. For example, it is not necessary to add vinegar to foods such as cabbage, beets, and cucumbers in order to preserve them. Since these vegetables have a high sugar content, they will naturally ferment and produce their own acid broth which will preserve them. Likewise milk ferments and acidifies readily, making products such as yogurt, kefir, and kwass. This sort of process also occurs in sour rye bread, where the sugars and starches in the grain ferment, producing lactic acid, and preserving the bread from the action of mold. In silos, lactic acid fermentation preserves grains from rotting, thus allowing the feed to be used throughout the winter. Several years ago I was searching an official government book to see if a product name I wanted to use on an herb formula was already used by another company. I had to laugh when I came across a trade name for a commercially-produced culture for starting the fermentation process of corn and other grains in silos, called "Silage-Mate."

Many traditional fermented beverages, such as yogurt, contain beneficial bacteria that improve digestion and help create an environment that is inhospitable for pathogenic microorganisms. These are often called "probiotics" to distinguish them from "antibiotics." Many scientific studies over the last 50 years have shown that probiotic organisms can improve the nutritional quality of foods, helping us to digest proteins and fats more efficiently. They can also help protect us from disease-causing organisms (like *Candida albicans*), boost our immune response, prevent diarrhea (for instance during radiation treatment), help prevent bowel cancer, aid in the body's detoxification process, lower cholesterol, and confer other healthy benefits. It is not clear whether the yeasts and bacteria in Kombucha have all of the same benefits, but they do produce some of the same constituents as *Lactobacillus acidophilus* and other commercially-available probiotic organisms.

Many practitioners of natural healing emphasize that digestion is truly the foundation of health. Digestion is our power center, the translator and regulator of our physical energy. Ultimately, the motive force or energy that fuels all life activities derives from the basic process called digestion. My feeling is that Kombucha tea with its friendly organisms and hydroxy acids has a beneficial effect on the digestive process.

Vinegar

The story of Kombucha is intimately related to the long history and human use of vinegar, because, as we have shown, many of the same organisms and biochemical reactions that are involved with the creation of vinegar go in to the making of Kombucha tea. It is likely to be the same process. In fact, if the Kombucha culture is left to work on the sugar and tea mixture too long, vinegar is produced.

Because vinegar is a natural result of wine and beer that has "aged" a little too long, it has probably been known and used by humans for at least 10,000 years. The first recorded mention of vinegar was about 5000 BC. The Babylonians write about the vinegar and wine that came from the dates they grew in abundance. The date trees were also tapped at the time of flowering to collect the sweet sap used in foods and allowed to ferment into palm wine, which is still made today in Saudi Arabia. The use of vinegar among the Babylonians was documented in their writings (Adams, 1985), and by the year 2000 BC, it became so popular as a condiment that a large commercial industry had sprung up.

Vinegar is an excellent solvent for essential oils and other flavor constituents of herbs, and the Babylonians also made use of spices such as garlic, tarragon, rue, saffron, and celery to add extra flavor, and for the purpose of strengthening the preservative effects of vinegar in the pickling process. This practice is still widely used today. Vinegar was also well-known in Mesopotamia between 3000 and 2000 BC, and Egyptian vinegar was considered the highest quality. Later it was highly prized by the Greeks and Romans, who were said to have a passion for vinegar.

Vinegar was also mentioned in the writings of the Assyrians, Greeks, and Romans as an important medicine in its own right, as well as the basis of a number of common foods and herbal preparations. They believed it to be astringent, to aid digestion, promote healthy liver and gall bladder function, as well as to refresh one and prevent scurvy (antiscorbutic) (Soyer, 1853).

The use of vinegar as a medicine probably reached its apogee in the school of Hippocrates, about 455 BC. The writings of Hippocrates are now thought to come from not only the man, but his followers and a number of other subsequent writers, collectively known as the Hippocratic school. The body of writing is called the "Hippocratic Corpus." Hippocrates was one of the first "natural healers" or holistic healers. I find it ironic that industrial or "modern" medicine has now taken Hippocrates as its ancestral mentor, even quoting the "Hippocratic Oath" as a basic tenet of their practice, when Hippocrates was really the "father of holistic medicine."

In Hippocratic writings, vinegar is mentioned many times. A blend of vinegar and honey, called "oxymel" (sour honey), was one of the most widely recommended remedies in the entire materia medica. Oxymel, or vinegar, formed the solvent to which many herbs were added in order to extract their active principles and aid in their assimilation by the body. Vinegar was generally considered cooling and drawing and was extolled for relieving such symptoms as vomiting of blood, itching of the skin, constipation, and was recommended for calming hysterical attacks, healing infected wounds and diphtheria (used as a steam inhalation), the dissipation of blood clots in the veins, and as a poultice, for cleaning out old sores.

Oxymel was highly regarded by Hippocrates, who says that it offers "manyfold benefits in acute illnesses...It moves the bowels, relieves respiration, especially when given warm and in moderation and when the mixture is not too sour, where it dampens the intestines; it sates the thirst, promotes release of gas and acts on the urine."

Furthermore, other ancient authors state that sour honey should be given warm in the summer and cold when there is great thirst, when it should first be mixed with water. It was popular as a drink to reduce fevers due to infected wounds (Dierbach, 1824).

The Jews used and wrote about vinegar extensively, both for cooking and as a healing substance. As a food, it was used as a condiment to be eaten with bread and staples and to preserve meat and vegetables. As a medicine, it was used as a hair rinse to cure dandruff (it is recommended for the same use today by herbalists), for toothaches, and as an antibacterial dressing for wounds.

Vinegar is mentioned in the Old Testament of the Bible many times, supporting its important cultural position as a food, medicine, and when diluted and sweetened, even as a drink. In fact, it is written that the last drink that Jesus took on the cross was a drink called posca (diluted vinegar), which was common to the Roman soldiers at the time of the crucifixion. The use of vinegar may have been introduced to Britain about the first century BC, and its use among the Celts was known. The word vinegar is of French origin, from *vin aigre* (sour wine).

Lemery, an alchemist who lived in the late 17th Century, in his *Course of Chymistry*, recommended a thick distilled vinegar, which he called "spirit of vinegar" to help the body "resist putrefaction," and says that it is "mixed with water...to stop hemorrhages taken inwardly, and to asswage inflammations applied outwrdly." He goes on to say precisely what constitutional type is best suited for the use of vinegar. "Neither vinegar, nor any other acids are proper for melancholy persons, because they mix the humoures [Ed: active fluids of the body] too much: They also turn those who take much of them lean; for they give too great consistency to the blood, and do hinder the chyle from distributing itself sufficiently through the body to give nourishment."

Although Kombucha is sometimes conjectured to originate in early Chinese history, it is possible that through its connection with the making of vinegar, it was known in ancient western cultures as well.

In China, vinegar is probably the seasoning known as "liu", which was written about as early as 1122 BC. In later centuries, it was extensively written about as an important condiment, used in major feasts and in everyday life. The importance of vinegar as a staple of the indigenous diet and as a preservative cannot be underestimated. It was extensively used to add flavor to foods, increase their nutritional value, perhaps by making minerals more bio-available to the body, and for pickling fish and other meats, and it continues to be used in a similar fashion today.

In Japanese culture, vinegar is at least as important a part of the culture as in China, perhaps more so. It was written about before the time of Christ and was said to have been brought from China to the southern part of Osaka in the period from 369 through 404 AD. A large-scale vinegar industry has been flourishing for over 300 years. Vinegar is an essential item in the Japanese household for making all manner of popular dishes. In particular, the manufacture of rice vinegar in Japan is very ancient. Kuroiwa Togo, one of Japan's leading proponents of this culturally important food, has a theory that vinegar made with rice has a higher percentage of free amino acids and acetic acid that makes it a healing drink for everyday use.

Among other claims, he asserts that it can help alleviate constipation, intestinal obstruction (when used as an injection), sinus infection, diluted as a rinse (10 ml of vinegar 50-50 with water) twice daily, as a rinse for eliminating dandruff, and as a health drink to help prevent arteriosclerosis (Togo, 1977).

Today, vinegar is used extensively all over the world, and the annual per capita consumption in industrialized countries is above 2 liters. In the United States, vinegar has a long history of folk-use for its healthful properties. Apple cider vinegar has been sold in health food stores since the 1950s and became quite popular as a home remedy, for everything from wounds to arthritis (Bragg and Bragg, n.d.).

Vinegar is antiseptic when applied topically to wounds and cuts; in a similar fashion, a cone of cotton dipped in vinegar and inserted into the ear is said to help heal outer ear infections (Diggs, 1989). Vinegar is also well-known as a domestic remedy to help alleviate the pain and inflammation of arthritis and rheumatism. Mugwort vinegar is widely recommended by herbalists of today for helping ease the inflammation and itching of poison oak rashes and other skin irritations. Rosemary and nettles macerated in vinegar make a cleansing hair rinse, which helps to fight dandruff.

Contemporary scientific studies of the health effects of consuming vinegar are scant. However, we can hypothesize, given what we know about acetic and other acids, that vinegar is antibacterial, that its acidity is helpful for digestion, and that, given its long historical healthful reputation, it may have other benefits. In one Japanese study, *in vivo* in mice, vinegar made from uncooked barley beer demonstrated a strong antitumor effect (Kubota et al, 1988).

Kombucha: Is It Safe?

Kombucha has its critics, and they generally have two objections to making the tea at home and consuming it on a regular basis. The first is the risk of contamination of Kombucha tea with dangerous pathogenic organisms. The second is the possibility of immune suppression or other undesirable effects from its purported antibiotic activity.

Probably the most vocal critic that I have encountered is Paul Stamets, a mushroom cultivator from Washington state. He became aware of Kombucha in 1980. In 1990, he sent it off to a lab (an interested drug company) to be tested for potential activity. The lab found a strong antibacterial effect from the tea—it was effective against antibiotic-resistant strains of *Staphylococcus aureus*, the bacteria responsible for "staph" infections, such as serious sore throats. The company wanted to investigate it further in the hopes that a marketable compound could be isolated, purified, and synthesized, possibly leading to other useful compounds. When Stamets informed them that the culture was not a single organism, but a community of different yeasts and bacteria, they were disappointed and wanted to charge him for the time they had "wasted" and expenses.

Stamets believes that because this lab had found a strong antibacterial activity from the tea, that it should not be taken on a daily basis, because it might have the same side effects as such purified antibiotics as penicillin, and it might lead to immune suppression. Natural medicine advocate Andrew Weil, MD, voices similar concerns. "It contains significant quantities of antibiotics, and that may be why it is beneficial, but that could induce further bacterial resistance. Overuse of antibiotic medicines is a major emerging problem, giving rise to new disease pathogens that are resistant to existing antibiotics, and individuals in whom antibiotics no longer are effective."

The other major concerns of Stamets and Weil involve contamination. Because people growing Kombucha tea at home don't usually have training in sterile lab technique, they may unwittingly allow pathogenic organisms to enter the brew and flourish. These organisms might produce toxic compounds or, in people with severely compromised immune systems, could lead to infections from ingesting them along with the tea. "My cultures spontaneously contaminated with poisonous molds," says Stamets. When one makes bread, or yogurt, the culture is semi-selective, he argues, whereas adding sugar to water enriched with nitrogen creates an environment "open to virtually every life form on this planet." Although "the organisms involved in Kombucha itself are not toxic," he says, "contamination is a big caveat." He says he has heard of cases of severe kidney pains, shortness of breath, and rashes. "I believe the danger to the public far outweighs any potential benefit at this time. I would hope that physicians would explore the potential uses of this colony of organisms, if prepared under clean-room conditions, and could present to the public information about who would benefit from drinking this fermented beverage. In my view, people now are sick and drinking it, may get sicker."

In Iowa, the death of one woman and the hospitalization of another, after drinking Kombucha tea, has prompted serious inquiry by the federal Centers for Disease Control and the federal Food and Drug Administration. The woman who died was a diabetic in her 60s, with several other health problems, who drank large amounts of the tea. The woman who survived was hospitalized with shortness of breath and cardiac failure and later recovered. She reported that the batch of Kombucha she drank was so vile she could hardly get it down, but she managed to do so, because she thought it was "good for her."

Stamets reports that there have been some cases of people with HIV who developed AIDS after drinking the tea. It is also possible that the protective effects from the beneficial organisms in Kombucha tea would have the opposite effect of retarding the growth of pathogens in such people, just as they do in the tea itself. For that matter, every person already harbors potentially pathogenic species, such as *Candida albicans*. It is just a question of ecological balance, coupled with immune status, emotional health, and many other factors.

The conjecture of the critics and the adverse reactions deserve further discussion. The determination of the safety of any herb or food is, of course, an important one. See the Resource Section on p.57 for commercially-brewed Kombucha sources.

Antibiotics — Or Antibacterial Biological Inhibitors?

The possibility that some powerful unknown antibiotic from the organisms in Kombucha could be harmful is unlikely, for the following reasons:

▸ The organisms are well-known and a number of studies on the compounds that they produce exist and are readily accessible.

▸ All of the organisms have been reported from traditional fermented foods used by millions of people over hundreds, if not thousands, of years with no reports of ill-effects that I can find in the literature, including a search of the Medlars database, the world's largest medical database.

▸ Science has identified several antibacterial compounds from fermented foods and from bacteria that occur in Kombucha. These include nisin (an antibacterial polypeptide, which belongs to a class of pathogenic inhibitors known as bacteriocins), acetic and lactic acids, and other organic acids and peroxides.

▸ Although nisin and similar bacteriocins such as *streptococcin A-FF22* and *diplococcin* are powerful inhibitors of bacteria, Hurst and Hoover (1993) have called them "biological inhibitors," and state that it is not justifiable to call them antibiotics. They are not presently used therapeutically, though there is increasing interest in them by scientists.

The authors conclude that because nisin is present in farmhouse cheese and milk, "it is likely that nisin or substances similar to it have been consumed for a significant length of time without apparent ill effects." Although nisin and similar compounds are unlikely to be harmful, even when taken long-term, they do inhibit pathogenic bacteria, such as *Clostridium botulinum* and *C. butyricum*, though its activity varies with the strain of pathogen, the pH of the environment (it works better in an acid environment like Kombucha tea), and other factors. In general, yeasts, molds, and gram negative bacteria are not affected. Nisin is especially effective for the preservation of pasteurized cheese products, and as such, it has been approved as a food additive in many European countries. Although nisin has not been identified from Kombucha yet, nisin-like compounds have been identified from many similar organisms to ones found in the Kombucha community.

Pathogenic Bacteria in an Acid Environment

The possibility that a home-brewed batch of Kombucha would become contaminated with pathogenic bacteria is also highly unlikely. One reason is the acidic nature of Kombucha tea. Pathogenic organisms are known to be sensitive to the pH of their environment. Some pathogenic organisms cannot grow in a medium that is too acid. Bacteria in particular tend to be more sensitive to acid conditions, and many are not able to survive in a pH under 4.5. Yeasts and molds have a wider range of tolerance, with molds being the most tolerant. This may partly explain why at a pH of 5.0-4.0, Kombucha tea will not support the growth of pathogenic bacteria, which tend to be among the most dangerous of the pathogenic organisms that would grow in such a medium. This is also why if there is any contamination in a batch of Kombucha tea it will probably be in the form of various molds. This, incidentally, is also Stamets' (1994-1995) view.

One current concept in food preservation is the "multiple-barrier" concept. This means that instead of using high concentrations of a bactericidal chemical to preserve a food, which is more likely to have harmful effects in humans, several compounds with much less potential toxicity are used in tandem with one another, thus effectively inhibiting potential pathogens in a food with less risk to human health.

Several tests for pathological organisms occurring in traditional fermented foods have consistently shown that they are safe, and samples tested were consistently free of aflatoxins, which are among the most toxic of fungal by-products (Frank, 1991; Hesseltine & Wang, 1986). Food scientists have taken a clue from the natural keeping qualities of traditional fermented foods and are starting to use bacteriocidins in conjunction with "acidulants" to mimic natural preservatives in foods. Commonly used acidulants include acetic acid, lactic acid, gluconic acid (monocarboxylic organic acids), all of which are found in Kombucha tea, and others (Doores, 1993). These organic acids all occur commonly in fermented and unfermented foods, and despite some reported side effects in animals and humans are generally considered safe for food use. Acetic acid has been reported to be one of the most effective at inhibiting a variety of potential food-borne pathogens (Doores, 1993), including *Salmonella enteritidis, E. coli, Bacillus spp.*, *Clostridium botulinum, Listeria monocytogenes, Pseudomonas aeruginosa*, yeasts and molds, and not just because of its acidity (Chung & Goepfert, 1970). In addition, it has one of the highest LD50 of any of the organic acids (4,960 mg/kg).

Kombucha tea usually contains from 0.5 to 3% acetic acid, depending on how long the culture is allowed to work on the alcohol and other constituents. This is mostly above effective antimicrobial levels. About 1% appears to be a good general concentration for inhibition of most pathogens (Doores, 1993), but as little as 0.1% of undissociated acetic acid will slow or stop the growth of most pathogenic food poisoning and spore-forming bacteria, and 0.3% will inhibit the growth of mycotoxigenic molds (Baird-Parker, 1980). Kombucha tea generally contains between 0.5 and 1.5% acetic acid.

Based on scientific tests, researchers have reported that only a very limited range of microorganisms can grow in vinegar. In a review of 84 samples of spoiled vinegar-preserved foods in the UK, the researchers found only *Lactobacillus spp.*, yeasts such as *Pichia membranaefaciens* and *Saccharomyces acidifaciens*, and *Moniliella acetoabutans*, a fungus that is apparently non-pathogenic, as the primary organisms of infection (Adams, 1985). I could find no mention of the latter species after a thorough search of toxline and Medlars and a review of several current texts on pathogenic microorganisms.

Acetic acid is found in such common foods as pickles, mustard, catsup, salad dressings, mayonnaise, and sausages. It is listed as "generally recognized as safe" (GRAS) by the FDA (21 CFR 184.1005). No daily maximum safe dose allowance is noted for acetic acid. Citric acid, found commonly in citrus fruits, and lactic acid, found in many traditional fermented foods such as sauerkraut, yogurt, and kefir, are also considered safe, and they have some antipathogenic properties, though not as strong as acetic acid. They occur in lesser amounts in Kombucha tea.

Yeast, at least commercial baker's yeast samples, has been extensively tested for contaminating organisms. It is grown in open fermenters and thus not under sterile conditions. The fermenting solution in which the yeast grows is less acidic (usually between pH 5 and 6 at the end of fermentation), so it is more likely that undesirable molds and other potentially pathogenic organisms will grow than in Kombucha tea, which also has a high yeast count, but a more acidic environment. Identified contaminants include bacteria from the genus *Leuconostoc*, *Lactobacillus*, which are mainly lactic-acid producers that are found in many traditional foods, also some coliform organisms, often *Aerobacter aerogenes* and occasionally some *E. coli.* The latter species can be pathogenic or not, depending on the strain. Wild yeasts are also commonly detected, such as *Candida utilis, Rhodotorula spp., Oidium lactis* or *Monilia spp.*, and occasionally *Saccharomyces paradoxus, Candida utilis, T. minor, C. krusei, C. mycoderma, C.krusei, C. tropicalis, Trichosporon cutaneum, Torulopsis candida,* and *Rhodotorula mucilaginosa.*

Yeasts contain significant amounts of nucleic acids in the form of RNA and DNA, which contribute to increased levels of uric acid found in the blood serum and urine of people who are fed high levels of the cells (45-135 g/day). Thus, people with problems of uric acid metabolism or who have gout should limit the use of yeast and yeast-containing products. The safe limit of food yeast in the average diet is estimated to be 30 grams/day. Yeast also contains histamine and tyramine (0.1-1.6 gm tyramine and 0.2-2.8 mg histamine per gram of yeast). A noticeable effect is seen on the blood pressure and pulse rate of people who eat high concentrations of yeast extracts, but this effect is probably minimal when less than 30 grams of whole yeast are consumed per day.

One of the most persuasive arguments in favor of the safety of making and using Kombucha at home is the fact that vinegar manufacturers make it on a large scale all over the world "quite satisfactorily without strict and costly sterility controls." The specific organisms involved in the process are of purely academic interest to the vinegar brewer since pure cultures are not widely employed in the industry. These quotes come from M.R. Adams, a researcher from the Tropical Development and Research Institute, Department of Microbiology, University of Surrey in the UK (Adams, 1985). In some Asian societies, often the vessels themselves, such as bamboo collection vessels of palm vinegar, act as an inoculating source of cultures for a new batch of vinegar. Often, a new batch is begun by adding a small amount of unpasteurized "mother" vinegar. This is a common practice in household production and is used commercially in Pakistan (Wahid & Chughtai, 1969) and, in particular, in Japan where about 60-70% of vinegar production is by surface culture techniques (Adams, 1985).

Although some critics caution against making the beverage at home or drinking Kombucha tea, it is certainly no more difficult than making yogurt or sauerkraut. As Günther Frank points out, the making of Kombucha has been successfully handed down from generation to generation by the Chinese for over 2000 years without any sterile lab techniques.

After a thorough search of the literature, careful consideration, and my own experience, I am inclined to give Kombucha a clean bill of health, if it is made properly with attention to cleanliness of hands and utensils. Preparing food and medicine with our own (clean!) hands certainly has its merits and eliminates the endless environmentally-unfriendly packaging we are constantly having to deal with. Of course, conditions vary, and as with any food preparation, there is always a chance that a batch could become contaminated. I would and do drink the tea myself, and I would have no problem recommending it to others, even my children. Each person must make their own choice based on available information and their own experience.

If there is a cause for concern, however, it is certainly the possibility of spontaneous contamination with molds. Stamets (1994-1995) reports that after experimenting with Kombucha he has observed spontaneous contamination of batches with various green, pink, or black molds. He is most concerned about *Aspergillus* molds, which he reports to contain water-soluble toxins that are highly carcinogenic, most likely aflatoxins. Fortunately, acetic acid is effective in stopping the production of aflatoxin by at least some *Aspergillus* spp. For instance, it can completely inhibit aflatoxin production by *Aspergillus parasiticus*, when concentrations are 1% or higher, and decrease their production by 70 and 90% respectively at concentrations of 0.6 to 0.8% (Doores, 1993).

Some *Aspergillus* spp. are helpful to humans and non-toxic, for instance *Aspergillus oryzae*, cultures of which are used to make rice koji in Japan (Hsu, 1989). Vinegar and acetic acid can also strongly inhibit the growth of some species of *Aspergillus*. For instance, acetic acid is known to inhibit the growth of *Aspergillus niger* and

A. flavus at levels as low as 0.4% (Masai, 1975; Spicher & Isfort, 1988). According to Bennet (1990), most species of *Aspergillus* are not a health threat when ingested, though they can cause immune reactions when their spores are inhaled. For the average person who has no severe immune deficiency conditions like AIDS, he suggests that there is no great concern: "The most important determinant of infection is the immune status of the patient, not the intensity of exposure." For this reason, he recommends that immuno-compromised individuals avoid unnecessary mold spore exposure.

Stamets is concerned that people making the tea at home would not know when a particular batch is contaminated with mold, and, if they did, might be tempted to simply "pull out the *Aspergillus* colonies with a fork," and drink the tea. He advises that if there is *any* indication of mold contamination ("most often the contaminants are green, pink or black mold-islands floating on the surface of the tea"), that one either discard it entirely, or carefully re-purify the tea. That can be done by removing a portion of the Kombucha mother, thoroughly washing it in cold water, and introducing it to a new batch of sugared tea. Stamets writes that a firm rubbery texture is a good indicator of whether the Kombucha organism has been degraded by infection from potential pathogens. If the organism falls apart when handled, it is best to discard it.

This is not new advice. In a 1957 article published in German, the authors (Steiger & Steinegger, 1957) note that "Henneberg (1926) mentions mold, moldy yeast, and extraneous vinegar bacteria...All these obtrusions can be removed by washing the fungus under running water."

We concur that such careful preparation is important. Common sense also dictates washing one's hands carefully before handling the culture, thoroughly cleaning and sterilizing the container to be used with boiling water, and not leaving the culture out of the fermentation container any longer than necessary. As an additional caution, one can add a small amount of cider vinegar or lemon juice to a new batch. As Steiger and Steinegger (1957) advise, "Since the extraneous germs often cannot handle acid as well as the organisms of the tea fungus community, Henneberg suggests to initially acidify the culture fluid somewhat, for example, using lemon, vinegar, or already prepared "Teekwass." Teekwaas is another name for Kombucha.

Is Kombucha for You?

Kombucha tea appears to be a traditional fermented beverage, which provides nutrition, especially B vitamins and some amino acids, has the ability to selectively retard the growth of potentially pathogenic bacteria, and may provide health benefits similar to other fermented foods and beverages, such as vinegar. It may also benefit digestion. Future studies, we hope, will establish whether it can play a role in any of the wide variety of illnesses that proponents now claim. It may do so. However, it is unlikely to be a panacea—a one-stop cure-all. In thousands of years, no such panacea has ever been found.

If you are immuno-compromised, HIV-positive, or a person with AIDS, it is best not to experiment with Kombucha tea until more is known about how a person with lowered immunity responds to this living beverage. Indeed, if you have any serious medical condition, such as cancer or diabetes, it is best to seek out a holistic-oriented health practitioner before embarking on a program with Kombucha tea.

It is also a good idea to start small. German researchers (Steiger & Steinegger, 1957) talk about doses of a few spoonfuls of the tea. If you have decided to add Kombucha to your daily routine and have secured a properly made clean batch, a reasonable daily amount to begin with would be two ounces, about a quarter of a cup. After a few weeks, you can increase that to half a cup (four ounces) with an upper limit of eight ounces a day.

One day, we may find that Kombucha tea lives up to some, or even many, of the health claims that its enthusiasts proclaim. It is our fervent hope that there will be contemporary studies to determine how it acts on the body, both in wellness and disease. Until then, we can enjoy this ancient, traditional fermented beverage, well-prepared, in reasonable amounts, as part of a lifestyle that includes a proper diet, exercise, and relaxation.

How to Make Kombucha Tea

Zeller (1924) warned against using alternative mixtures of tea or sugar, as substitutions can disrupt the delicate balance of yeasts and bacteria. The Swiss pharmacist, Bergold, also cautioned against using older fungi, which might be contaminated by various molds. Apparently cultures of dubious origin exist on the market.

1. Pour 34 oz of water into a glass or enamel pan and set on stove

2. As the water is heating up, add 2 oz sugar and stir until dissolved.

3. When the water begins to boil, remove the pan from the heat and add 1-4 teaspoons or 2-5 teabags (to taste) of either black or green tea. Steep 10-15 minutes. Be careful not to let the water boil for more than a moment or two; if the sugar is overheated, compounds called hydroxymethylfurfural are produced, which can inhibit the growth of many yeasts.

4. If tea leaves have been used, strain through a strainer; if a teabag was used, remove it.

5. Let the mixture cool to lukewarm and then pour it into a glass jar or glazed earthenware jar; to make larger amounts use a large glass cooking bowl or a glass aquarium (Frank, 1991). Ideally the container should have a wide mouth, and there shouldn't be too much air space above the liquid.

6. Add about 10% Kombucha from the previous batch (if you are making it for the first time, get the extra starter liquid with the culture, or add two tablespoons of boiled vinegar to the tea).

7. Place the culture in the liquid, taking care to not break the layer on the upper surface (the smooth, shiny surface should be face up, with the brown, rougher layer underneath). Sometimes the culture floats and sometimes it sinks to the bottom, which may depend on how soft or hard the water is.

8. Use cheesecloth to cover the mouth of the container and secure with a rubber band.

9. Place in a warm spot, and leave without moving it for 8-10 days*. The optimal temperature range for Kombucha culture is approximately 70-77 Fahrenheit, though it will also grow from 83 to 89. If the temperature is too low, the metabolic processes of the bacteria slow down, which might make the culture more prone to the growth of molds. If too high, volatile flavor components are lost, leading to an inferior tea. It will grow poorly or not at all when the temperature is much below 65 degrees or above 90 degrees.

10. Keep out of direct sunlight. The bacteria work better in the semi-dark. The vitality of the vinegar bacteria is said to be reduced by direct exposure to light. Violet light will affect them the most, and red light, very little (Mitchell, 1926).

11. The surface of the mother should be in contact with an ample supply of air. Cover the culture with a layer of cheesecloth or loosely-woven cloth to allow free flow of air and still keep out the light. The formation and growth of the zoogleal body, or pellicle, produced by *A. aceti subsp. xylinum* are said to be promoted by a condition of high oxygen. The pellicle may increase the access to oxygen that the vinegar bacteria need in order to thrive, by suspending them in it at the surface of the fermenting vinegar. More air will encourage the growth of the mother; less air will inhibit its growth. When there is a severe shortage of oxygen, undesirable contaminating organisms may grow, such as molds. (We covered one of our Kombucha cultures with a thick cloth, and soon we had a nice crop of blue-green mold growing all over the mother).

12. Measure the pH of the fermenting liquid at various intervals. A healthy culture will maintain an optimum pH of between 4.5 and 6.0. Testing strips can be purchased at many drugstores.

13. After the batch is ready, wash your hands carefully, then remove the culture (the "Kombucha mother").

14. Strain the tea into bottles and store in the refrigerator or in another cool place. Because there may be some carbonation, don't fill the bottle all the way up to the top; Frank (1991) suggests using corks rather than caps in case pressure builds up. If a "sparkling" beverage is desired, you can actually use old champagne bottles, tying down the top, but be cautious when taking the top off.

15. Leave the yeast sediment in the original container, but once a month it should be poured out as well and the container washed with boiling hot water. At this time, wash the culture with cold water and then replace it in the container, once it has cooled somewhat.

16. Keep approximately 10% of the tea in the fermentation container (unless it needs to be washed, in which case it may be poured back in after the container is washed).

17. Do not smoke in the same room where the Kombucha is growing; reportedly, smoking can cause molds to form or the Kombucha mother to dissolve. (Of course, if you smoke, finding a way to stop is the most positive health action you can take).

18. Kombucha can be made from many bases, including herbal tea and fruit juice, or honey instead of sugar, but we do not recommend it until more is known about the safe preparation of the tea. In particular, essential oils from a number of spices, such as cinnamon and fennel, strongly retard the growth of yeasts. The high tannin content of black tea, for example, may be one factor in keeping pathogens from growing on the mother or in the tea itself. If the small amount of caffeine in the final product is a concern, green tea will work. It contains a higher amount of inhibitory tannins than black tea, with less free caffeine.

19. If molds form (often in the form of of blue, green, red or black floating islands), discard the tea, and remove the Kombucha mother. Bring it under a cold water faucet; if the pellicle tears easily or seems to be disintegrating, throw it out. Otherwise, wash it carefully under cold running water, place it aside, and begin to make the tea again from scratch. Sterilize the containers by filling with boiling water, then washing. Some authors (de Silva and Saravanapavan, 1969) suggest that when a mother becomes contaminated with mold, one should wash it gently with water, rubbing it off with the finger, then rinse in pure apple cider vinegar.

20. When in doubt, throw it out.

21. If you have extra Kombucha mothers, or "babies", pass them on!

22. Be careful where you discard Kombucha mothers. Reportedly, they can grow in septic systems, even in municipal sewers. So do not flush them down the toilet or dispose of them down the kitchen sink. Throw them in the garbage or bury them with appropriate ceremony.

* Some people contend the tea should be poured off after 6 days in winter and after 3-4 days in summer, when it should be allowed to sit in glass containers for another 3 days before drinking. Frank (1991) writes that after 12-14 days, the sugar is completely converted and the taste similar to dry wine—and it is easier to digest at this stage. Also, Russian researchers have reported that the antibiotic activity found in Kombucha is at its highest peak on the 7th and 8th days (Frank, 1991).

References

Adams, M.R. 1985. Vinegar. In *Microbiology of Fermented Foods*, vol. 1, B.J.B. Wood (Ed.). New York: Elsevier.

Ayres, J.C. et al. 1980. *Microbiology of Foods*. San Francisco: W.H. Freeman and Co.

Baird-Parker. 1980. Organic acids. In *Microbial Ecology of Foods*, Vol. 1, Factors Affecting Life and Death of Microorganisms, Int. Com. Microbiol Spec. Foods (Ed.). New York: Academic Press.

Bennet, J.E. 1990. *Aspergillus* spp. In *Principles and Practice of Infectious Diseases*. New York: Curchill Livingston, Inc.

Bragg, P.C. and P. Bragg. *The Miracle of Apple Cider Vinegar*. n.d. Santa Barbara: Health Science.

Brannt, W.T. 1914. *A Practical Treatise on the Manufacture of Vinegar*. Philadelphia: Henry Carey Baird & Co.

Buchanan, R.E. and N.E. Gibbons (eds.). 1974. *Bergey's Manual for Determinative Bacteriology*, 8th ed. Baltimore: The Williams & Wilkins Co.

Chung, K.C. and J.M. Goepfert. 1970. Growth of *Salmonella* at low pH. *J. Food Sci.* 35: 326-8.

Conner, H.A. and R.J. Allgeier. 1976. Vinegar: Its history and development. *Adv. appl. Microbiol.* 20:81-133.

Cook, A.H. (ed.). 1958. *The Chemistry and Biology of Yeasts*. New York: Academic Press.

De Vincenzi, M. et al. 1987. Volatile compounds in food. In *Food Additives and Contaminants*. New York: Taylor and Francis.

de Silva, R.L. and T.V. 1968. Sarravanapavan. Tea cider—a potential winner. *The Tea Quarterly* 39:37-41.

Dierbach, J.H. 1824. *The Medicinal Plants of Hippocrates*. Translated by S. Coble and C. Hobbs, 1994. Publication in progress.

Diggs, L.J. 1989. *Vinegar*. San Francisco: Quiet Storm Trading Co.

Doores, S. Organic Acids. 1993. In Davidson, P.M. and A.L. Branen (eds.), *Antimicrobials in Foods*. New York: Marcel Dekker, Inc.

Fasching, R. (1985) 1994. *Tea Fungus Kombucha: The Natural Remedy and its Significance in cases of Cancer and Other Metabolic Diseases*. Steyr, Austria: Wilhelm Ennsthaler.

Frank, G.W. 1991. *Healthy Beverage and Natural Remedy from the Far East*. Steyr, Austria: Wilhelm Ennsthaler.

Flück, V. and E. Steinegger. 1957. A new yeast from the tea mushroom. *Scientia Pharmaceutica* 25:43-44.

Freydberg, N. and W.A. Gortner. 1941. *The Food Additives Book*. New York: Bantam Books, pp. 553-54.

Gadd, C.H. 1933. Tea Cider. *Tea Quarterly* 6:48-53.

Gallardo-de Jesus, E. et al. 1971. A study on the isolation and screening of microorganisms for production of diverse-textured nata. *The Philippine Journal of Science* 100:41-49.

Gálvez, M.C. et al. 1994. Analysis of polyphenolic compounds of different vinegar samples. *Z. Lebensm. Untes. Forsch.* 199:29-31.

Godfrey, A. 1985. Production of Industrial Enzymes and Some Applications in Fermented Foods. In Wood, B.J.B., *op. cit.*

Greenshields, R.N. 1975. Malt vinegar manufacture (Part 1). *The Brewer* (July):295-98.

Hauser, S.P. 1990. Dr. Sklenar's Kombucha mushroom infusion—a biological cancer therapy. *Schweiz Rundsch. Med. Prax.* 79:243-46.

Hesseltine, C.W. and H.L. Wang. 1986. *Indigenous Fermented Food of Non-Western Origin.* Berlin: J. Cramer.

Holt et al. 1994. *Bergey's Manual of Determinative Bacteriology.* Baltimore: Williams and Wilkins Co.

Hsu, E.J. 1989. Automated method for a semi-solid fermentation used in the production of ancient quality rice vinegar and/or rice wine. United States Patent.

Hurst, A. and D.G. Hoover. 1993. Nisin. In Davidson and Branen, *op. cit.*

Jay, J.M. 1992. *Modern Food Microbiology.* New York: Van Nostrand Reinhold (An Avi Book).

Kreger-Van Rij, N.J.W. (ed.). 1984. *The Yeasts, a taxonomic study,* 3rd ed. Amsterdam: Elsevier Science Publishers.

Kubota, T. et al. 1988. Antitumor activity of vinegar made from pearl barley grain. Nippon. *Nogeikagaku Kaishi* 62:23-28.

Kwanashie, H.O. 1989. Screening of 'kargasok tea' I: anorexia and obesity. *Biochemical Society Transactions* 17:1132-3.

Lapuz, M.M. et al. 1967. The nata organism—cultural requirements, characteristics, and identity. *The Philippine Journal of Science* 96:91-108.

List, P.H. and L. Hörhammer. 1973. *Hagers Handbuch der Pharmazeutischen Praxis,* 7 vols. New York: Springer-Verlag.

List, P.H. and W. Hufschmidt. 1959. The Biogenic Amines and Amino Acids of the Tea Mushroom. *Pharmazeutische Zentralhalle* 98:593-98.

Mitchell, C.A. 1926. *Vinegar: Its Manufacture and Examination.* London: Charles Griffin and Co., Ltd.

Mollison, B. 1993. *The Permaculture Book of Ferment and Human Nutrition.* Tyalgum, Australia: Tagari Publications.

Nakayama, S. et al. 1980. Utilization of slimy polysaccharide produced by acetic acid bacteria. *Nippon Shokuhin Kogyo Gakkaishi* 27:377-80.

Phaff, H.J. et al. 1978. *The Life of Yeasts.* London: Harvard University Press.

Prescott, S.C. and C.G. Dunn. 1959. *Industrial Microbiology.* New York: McGraw-Hill Book Co., Inc.

Reed, G. And H.J. Peppler. 1973. *Yeast Technology.* Westport, CT: Avi Publishing Co.

Reiss, J. 1994. Influence of different sugars on the metabolism of the tea fungus. *Z. Lebensm. Unters. Forsch.* 198:258-61.

Rose, A.H. and J.S. Harrison. 1987. *The Yeasts* (2 vols.). New York: Academic Press.

Rosebury, Theodor. 1962. *Microorganisms Indigenous to Man.* New York: McGraw-Hill Book Co.

Ross, P. et al. 1991. Cellulose biosynthesis and function in bacteria. *Microbiological Reviews* 44:35-58.

Soyer, A. 1853. *The Pantropheon or History of Food and its Preparation.* London: Simpkin, Marshall and Co.

Stadelmann, V.E. 1907. About Tea Mushroom. A Literature Summary. *Sydowia* XI, 1/6.

Stamets, P. 1995. My Adventures with the Blob. *Mushroom the Journal* Winter, 1994-5: 5-9.

Steiger, K.E. and E. Steinegger. 1957. On the Tea Fungus. *Pharmaceutica Acta Helvetiae* 32(4):133-54.

Steinkruas, K.H. 1985. Bio-enrichment: Production of Vitamins in Fermented Foods. In Wood, *op. cit.*

Togo, K. 1977. *Rice Vinegar.* Tokyo: Kenko Igakusha Co., Ltd.

Utkin, L.M. 1937. A new microorganism of the Acetobacter group. *Microbiology* (U.S.S.R.) 6:433-4.

Vincenzi et al. 1987. Volatile compounds in food. In *Food Additives and Contaminants*, Vol. 4. New York: Taylor & Francis.

Wahid, M.A. and M.I.D. Chughtai. 1969. Studies in the chemical activities of microorganisms. VII: Acetic acid (Vinegar) from indigenous raw materials. *Pak. J. Scientific Res.* 21:88-93.

Williams, W.S. and R.E. Cannon. 1989. Alternative environmental roles for cellulose produced by *Acetobacter xylinum. Applied and Environmental Microbiology* 55:2448-52.

Wood, B.J.B. and M.M. Hodge. 1985. Yeast-Lactic acid bacteria interactions and their contribution to fermented foodstuffs. In Wood, *op. cit.*

Additional References

(Note: This bibliography has been included to show the cultural context and to demonstrate how much discussion has been generated on the topic of Kombucha over the last 100 years. The references are cited in chronological order.)

Kombucha —
A Bibliography from Europe, 1852-1957

(German titles translated by C. Hobbs)

Thomson, R.D. 1852. The nature and chemical effects of the mother of vinegar. *Ann. Chem. Pharm.* 83, 89-93.

Brown, A.J. 1896. On an Acetic Ferment which forms Cellulose. *J. Chem. Soc. Transactions.* (London) 49, 432-439.

Brown, A.J. 1887. Note on the Cellulose formed by *Bacterium Xylinum. J. Chem. Soc. Transactions.* (London) 51, 643.

Kobert, R. 1896. About Kwass. Its introduction into Western Europe. *Histor. Studien a. d. Pharmakol.* Inst. Univ. Dorpat 5, 100-131.

Bacinskoj, A.A. 1911. K Morfologij I biologij *Bacterium xylinum.* Brown, Russkij Vrae (St. Petersburg) 10 (51) 2104-2108, (The morphology and biology of *Bacterium xylinum* Brown.)

Saito, K. 1911. Technically-important East-Indian mushrooms. *Mikrokosmos* 5, (7) 145-150.

Bacinskoj, A.A. 1913. O tak' naz'ivaemom' manezursco-japonskom' gribe I cajnom kvase. Vracebnaja gazeta (Petrograd) 20 (30) 1063-1064. "About the so-called Manchurian-Japanese mushroom and Tee-Kwass. Referat: Zamkow, N.: 1914.)

Kobert, R. 1913. Der Kwass. A harmless low-cost people's drink, Halle a. d. S.: Tausch & Grosse. 2. Aufl. 82 S.

Bacinskaja, A.A. 1914. O rasprostranenii "cajnago kwasa" I *Bacterium xylinum* Brown. *Zurnal' mikrobiologii* (Petrograd) 1, (1, 2) 73-85. (The spread of "Tea-Kwass" and *Bacterium xylinum* Brown).

Zamkow, N. 1914. Referat: Batschinski, A.A. 1913. Russian Tea-vinegar. The so-called Manchurian-Japanese mushroom and Tea kwass. *Dtsch. Essigindustrie* 18, (28), 330-331.

Bazarewski, S. 1915. About the so-called Miracle Mushroom in the Baltic Provinces. *Korrblatt Naturforsch-Vereins Riga* 57, 61-80. Ref.: Matouschek, F. (1922).

Kobert, R. 1917. Tea kvass. *Mikrokosmos*, 11, (9), 159. (Kleine Mittellung).

Lindner, P. 1917. Tea kwass and the Tea kwass mushroom. *Mikrokosmos*, 11, (6), 93-98; vgl. auch Lindner, P.: 1918.

Lindner, P. 1918. Tea kwass and the Tea kwass mushroom. *Dtsch. Essigindustrie* 22, (48), 273-274; (49) 278-280; (50) 284-285. (Abdruck aus: *Mikrokosmos* 11, 93-98 (1917).

Matouschek, F. 1922. Referat: Bazarewski. S. The so-called "Miraculous mushroom" in the Baltic Province. (1915). *Zbl. Bakteriol.* II 55, 320-321.

Lind, J. 1925. En ganske ny Form af Medicin. *Arch. Pharmaci og Chemi.* (Kobenhaven) 32, 336.

Hennebert, W. 1926. *Handbook of fermentative bacteriology.* 2. Bd. p. 70 225, 379. Berlin: Paul Parey. 2. Aufl. 403 S.

Lzn. 1926. (Fragekasten-Antwort) " *Apoth. Ztg.* 41, (57) 771.

Anonymous. 1927. About Kombucha. *Sudetendeutsche Apothekerzig.* S. (38), 317-318.

Anonymous. 1927. (Fragekasten-Anfrage). *Die Umschau* 31, (50) 2 Beilagenseite.

B.v.P. 1927. (Fragekasten-Anfrage) *Prakticky lekaf* (Praha) 7, (3) 115.

Dinslage, E. and W. Ludorff. 1927. The "Indian tea mushroom." *Z. Unters. Lebensmittel* 53, 458-467.

Dubowitz, H. 1927. A "japan gomba". *Gyogyaszai* (Budapest) 67, (12) 274-275, (13) 303-304. (Der japanische Pilz.)

F.S. 1927. (Fragekasten-Anfrage) *Ars medici* 17, 538.

Harms, H. 1927. The Japanese tea mushroom. *Therapeut. Berichte* (Leverkusen) 1927, (12) 498-500.

Heider, N. 1927. (Fragekasten-Antwort). *Ars medici* 17, 605.

Heubner, W. 1927. *Otto Heubners Lebenschronik,* 228. Berlin: J. Springer. 228 S.

Irrgang, J. 1927. (Fragekasten-Antwort). *Ars medici* 17, 605.

Lederer, N. 1927. The Japanese Mushroom. *Biologische Heilkunst* (Dresden) 8, 579.

Lepa, H. 1927. (Fragekasten-Antwort) *Ars medici* 17, 655.

Lüwenheim, H. 1927. The Indian tea mushroom. *Apoth. Zig.* 42, (11) 148-149.

Müllerová, L. 1927. Kombucha. *Casopis ceskoslovenskeho Lekarnietva* 7, (4) 58-59.

Müllerová, N. 1927. "Japonska houba." (Fragekasten-Antwort). *Prakticky lekar* (Praha) 7, (3) 119.

Rosenbaum, J. 1927. Kombucha. *Practicky lekar* (Praha) 7, (15) 604.

Waldeck, H. 1927. The tea mushroom. *Pharm. Zentralhalle* 68, 789-790.

Anonymous. 1928. Prohibition of the Japanese mushroom "Kombucha." *Sudetendeutsche Apothekerzig.* 9, (2) 4. (Rubrik: "Amtliche Nachrichten").

Anonymous, 1928. The Kombucha Question. *Sudetendeutsche Apothekerzig.* 9, (10) 95-96.

Anonymous. 1928. Advertising the Japanese Mushroom Kombucha and its Preparations. *Sudetendeutsche Apothekerzig.* 9, (11) 105. (Rubrik: "Amtliche Nachrichten").

Anonymous. 1928. Kombucha-drink. (Questions and answers). *Dtsch. Essigindustrie* 32, (38) 333-334.

Anonymous. 1928. Effects of the Indian Tea Mushroom. *Drogisten-Zeitung* (Leipzig) 54, (52) 1499-1500.

Bing, M. 1928. Health effects of the "Kombucha mushroom". *Die Umschau* 32, (45) 913-914.

Bing, M. 1928. The Symbionts *Bacterium xylinum—Schizosaccharomyces Pombe* as a medicinal agent. *Die medizinische Welt*, 2 (42) 1576-1577.

Eberding, W. 1928. The Japanese Tea Mushroom. Volksheil (Berlin) 5, (5) 123-124.

Gince, V. 1928. Japnoskij gribok. *Gigiena pitanija* (Leningrad). 1928. (1) 15.

Gl. 1928. Teepilz (Questions-Answers). *Dtsch. Eddigindustrie* 32, (47) 413-414.

Harms, H. 1928. The Japanese or Indian Tea Mushroom. *Xrztlicher Wegweiser* (Berlin) 4. (17) 330.

Harms, H. 1928. The Japanese Tea Mushroom. *Pharmaz. Ber.* 3, (1) 1-3.

Lakowitz, N. 1928. The Tea Mushroom and Tea Kvass. *Apoth. Ztg.* 43, (19) 298-300.

Mollenda, L. 1928. Kombucha, its significance for health and and cultivation. *Dtsch. Essigindustrie* 32, (27) 243-244.

Rywosch, S. 1928. Kombucha, a new drink. *Die Umschau* 32, (30) 610, 614.

Rywosch, S. 1928. (short communication) The Japanese Tea Mushroom and Arteriosclerosis. *Die Weisse Fahne* (Pfullingen, Wurttemberg) 9, (2) 60.

Rywosch, S. 1928. The "Japanese Tea Mushroom." *Die Weisse Fahne* (Pfullingen, Wurtemberg) 9, (4) 184-185.

Saccardo, P.A. 1928. *Medusomuyces Gisevii*. Sylloge Fungorum 24, sect. II, 1314. Avellino (Italien): Coheredum Saccardo. 1438 S.

Steinmann, A. 1928. The Indian "Tea Mould." *De Bergcultures* (Djakarta) 2, II. 1113-1114.

Valentin, H. 1928. The usability of the Indian tea mushroom and its extraction in dried form. *Apoth. Zig.* 48, (101) 1533-1536.

W., 1928. Teekwass. (Fragekasten-Antwort). *Dtsch. Essigindustrie* 32, (17) 146-147.

Wiechowski, W. 1928. Which position should doctors take on the Kombucha-question? *Beitr. arzt. Fortbildg.* 6, (1) 2-10. (Referat: Molitor, H. 1929).

Anonymous. 1929. Fungojapon. *Pharm. Zentralhall.* 70, (17) 267. (Anmerkung: Rubrik: Chemie and Pharmazie).

Arauner, A. 1929. The Japanese tea mushroom. *Dtsch. Essigindustrie* 33, (2) 11-12.

Bing, M. 1929. About the "Kombucha Question." *Die Umschau* 33, (6) 118-119.

Gutmann, C. and H. Kallfelz. 1929. The clinical value of an oral antidiabetic medicine. *Klin. Woehenschr.* 8, 2246-2247.

Haehn, H. and M. Engel. 1929. The synthesis of lactic acid by *Bacterium xylinum*. Lactic acid fermentation by Kombucha. *Z. Bakt. Parasitenkde. and Infektionskrahkh.* 2 Abt. 79, 182-185.

Harms, H. 1929. The Tea Mushroom, Mo-Gu. *Chem. Zbl.* 1929, 11, 602. (Rubrik: Pharmazie, Spezialitaten und Geheimmittel).

Hermann, S. 1929. The synthesis of gluconic acid and keto-gluconic acid by *Bacterium gluconicum*, *Bacterium xylinum* and *Bacterium xylinoides*. *Biochem. Z.* 214, 357-367.

Hermann, S. 1929. Pharmacological investigations on the so-called Kombucha and its influence on the toxic effects of Cholecalciferol [naturally-occurring vitamin D]. *Klin. Wochenschr.* 8, 1752-1757.

Lakowitz, N. 1929. Teekwass. *Der Naturforscher* 5, (1) 18-19.

Martell, P. 1929. The Tea Mushroom as a Medicine. *Pharm. Zentralhalle* 70, 615-618.

Molitor, H.. 1929. Referat. Wiechowski, W.: Which position should the doctor take on the Kombucha-question? (1928). *Die tagliche Praxis* (Wien) 1, (2) 43-44.

Obst, W. 1929. Banana vinegar and the Tea mushroom. *Dtsch. Essigindustrie* 33, (18) 145-146.

Propfe, P. 1929. Kombucha. *Die Umschau* 33, (6) 118.

Floresco, N. 1930. Kombucha, A Psychological Study. *Bull. Fac. Stiinte Cernautl.* (Rumanien) 4, (1) 146-156.

Floresco, N. 1930. Tadpoles Nourished by Kombucha. *Bull. Fac. Stiinte Cernauti.* (Rumanien) 4, (1) 157-158.

Floresco, N. und A. Rafailesco-Floresco. 1930. Kombucha. Influence on the Development of Frog Eggs. *Bull. Fac. Cernauti.* (Rumanien) 4, (1) 159-163.

Floresco, N. 1930. Kombucha. Influence on the Development of the Tadpole. *Bull. Fac. Stiinte Cernauti.* (Rumanien) 4, (2) 220-226.

Floresco, N. 1930. Kombucha. Influence on the Isolated Heart. *Bull. Fac. Stiinte Cernauti.* (Rumanien) 4, 252-254.

Frank, N. 1930. Referat: Gutmann, C. u. H. Kalifelz. The clinical value of an oral antidiabetic remedy (1929), *Chem. Zbl.* I. 1489.

Hermann, S. 1930. The pharmacology of gluconic acid. A contribution to the problem of the effects of free acids in the organism. Part I. *Naunyn-Schmiedebergs Arch. exp. Pathol. u. Pharm.* 154, 43-160.

Hermann, S. 1930. Zur Pharmakologie der Gluconsaure. The pharmacology of gluconic acid. A contribution to the problem of the effects of free acids in the organism. Part 2. *Naunyn-Schmiedebergs Arch. exp. Pathol. u. Pharm.* 154, 43-160.

Hermann, S. 1930. The pharmacology of gluconic acid. A contribution to the problem of the effects of free acids in the organism. Part 3. *Naunyn-Schmiedebergs Arch. exp. Pathol. u. Pharm.* 154, 175-192.

Valentin, H. 1930. Primary active components of fermentation products from mushroom-extracted home drinks, as well as its spread. *Apoth. Ztg.* 45, (91) 1464-1465; (92) 1477-1478.

Anonymous. 1931. Kombucha, the Miracle Mushroom, Japanese tea mushroom, Tea mushroom. In: *Der Grosse Brockhaus*, Bd. 10, 346. Leipzig: F.A. Brockhaus.

Floresco, N. 1931. Chamboucho. Ferment solubles. *Bull. Fac. Stiinte Cernauti* (Rumanien) 5 (1) 1-14.

Hermann, S. and P. Neuschui. 1931. The biochemistry of vinegar bacteria and a proposal for a new systematic treatment. *Biochem. Z.* 283, 129-216.

Hermann, S. and The Pharmaceutical Works "Norgine" A.G. in Prague 1931: The process of the manufacture of effective therapeutic preparations with help from Kombucha. D.R. Patentschr. Nr. 538 028.

Schreyer, R. 1931. Comparative investigations on the synthesis of gluconic acid from the "mold mushroom." *Biochem. Z.* 240, 295-325.

Scerbacev, D.M. 1931. Cajn'ij ili japonski grib I ego problema. *Sovetskaja Farmacija* (5-6), 28-29. (The Tea Mushroom or Japanese Mushroom and Its Transformation).

Anonymous. 1932. Tea beer: A new use for tea. *Tea and Coffee Trade J.* (New York), August, 180, 182.

Anonymous. 1932. Tea-Cider. A new Drink in Java. *Tea Quarterly* (Talawakelle, Ceylon) 5, 126-127.

Anonymous. 1932. "Theebier". Mooie perspectieven vor groot binnen-v. *Nederlandsch-Indie* 16, (48) 1280-1281.

Anonymous. 1932. (Kurze Notiz) Alg. Landbouwweekbi. v. *Nederlandsch-Indie* 16, (46) 1223-1225.

Hermann, S. and P. Neuschul. 1932. Lactic acid- and pyruvic acid-synthesis from vinegar bacteria. *Biochem. Z.* 246, (4/6) 446-459.

Koolhaus, D.R. 1932. "Thea beer". Alg. Landbouwweekbl. v. *Nederlandsch-Indie* 16, (48) 1295.

Koolhaas, D.R. and K. Boedijn. 1932. (Rundschreiben). The tea-mushroom. *De Bergcultures* (Djakarta) 6, 259-260.

Koolhaas, D.R. and K. B. Boedijn. 1932. De "Tea Mushroom" in Nederlandsch-Indie. Voorlopige Mededeeling. *De Bergcultures* (Djakarta) 6, 299-303.

Gadd, C.H. 1933. Tea Cider. *Tea Quarterly.* (Talawakelle, Ceylon) 6, 48-53.

Barsha, J. and H. Hibbert. 1934. Studies on reactions relating to carbohydrates and Polysaccharides. XLVI. Structure of the cellulose synthesized by the action of *Acetobacter xylinus* on Fructose and Glycerol. *Canad. J. Res.* 10, 170-179.

Hermann, S. and P. Neuschul. 1934. The biochemistry of vinegar bacteria. A characteristic difference of *Bacterium gluconicum* (Hermann) from other vinegar bacteria concerning the influence of galactose. *Biochem. Z.* 270, (1/3) 6-14.

Hermann, S. and N. Fodor. 1935. C-Vitamin (1-Ascorbic acid-) production from a symbiosis of vinegar bacteria and yeasts. *Biochem. Z.* 276, (5/6), 323-325.

Hermann, S. and P. Neuschul. 1936. The oxydation of glucose from *Bacterium gluconicum* Hermann. *Biochem. Z.* 287, (5/6) 400-404.

Gordienko, M. 1937. Referat: Utkin, L.: A new microorganism from the group of vinegar bacteria. (1937). *Zbl. Bakt.* 98 II, 359).

Kasevnik, L.D. 1937. Biochimija Vitamina C. Soobstenie III. O sposobnosti japonskogo cajnogo griba sintezirovat Vitamin C. Bjull. exp. Biol. I Med. (Moskva) 3, (1) 87-88. (The Biochemistry of Vitamin C:3. The ability of the Japanese Tea Mushroom to synthesize vitamin C.) Referat: Schwaihold, N.: 1937.

Schwaibold, N. 1937. Referat: Kasevnik. L.D.: (The Biochemistry of Vitamin C: III. The capacity of the Japanese tea mushroom to synthesize Vitamin C.) 1937. *Chem. Zbl.*

Utkin, L. 1937. O novon microorganizme iz grupp'j uksusn'ih bakterij. *Mikrobiologija* (Moskva) 6, (4) 421-434. (About new microorganisms from the vinegar bacteria group.) Referat: Gordienko, M.: 1937.

Bernhauer, K. 1938. The biochemistry of the vinegar bacteria. Erg. Enzymforschg. 7, 246-280.

Kasevnik. L.D. 1940. O Nekotor'ih biohimiceskih osobennostjah t.n. cajnogo griba. Sbornik irudov Archangel'skij gosudarstven'ij Medicinskij Inst. 5, 116-121. (A biochemical peculiarity of the so-called tea mushroom. Heft des Med. Inst. Archangelsk No. 5).

Subov, M.I. 1947. K voprosu o znacenii nastoja tak naz'ivaemogo "cajnogo griba" kak terapevticescogo sredstva. Vrac. delo (Charkov) 27, (6) 511-512. (The significance of tea on the so-called "Tea mushroom" as a therapeutic agent."

Sakarjan, G.A. and L. T. Danielova. 1948. Antibiotieeskie svojstva nastoja griba *Medusomyces gisevi* (cajnogo griba). Soobstenie. 1. Trud'i Erevanskogo zooveterinariogo Instituta, 10, 33-45. (The significance of antibiotic of the liquid substance from *Medusomyces gisevii* (tea mushroom).

Fedorow, M.V. 1949. *Mikrobiologija*. Moskva: Gos. izdatel'stvo sel'skohoz. literatur'i. 236.

Mühietaler, K. 1949. The Structure of Bacterial Cellulose. *Biochim. et Biophys.* Acta 8, 527-535.

Naumova, E.K. 1949. Meduzin—Novoe antibioticeskoe vestestvo, Avtoreferat. Kazan'. (Medusin—a new antibiotic substance.)

Sakarjan, G.A. and L.T. Danielova. 1949. Lecebn'ie svojstva cajnogo griba (*Medusomyces gisevi*). *Veterinarija* (Moskva) 26, (10) 48-49. (The curative power of the tea mushroom.)

Vasil'kov, B.P. 1950. O "Cajnom gribe". *Priroda* (Leningrad). 39, (7) 59-60.

Rentz, N. 1951. Referat: Tindimnik, V. S. S. E. Funk and I. V. Sabinskaja. The question of the therapeutic vinegar bacteria therapeutic quality of the tea mushroom. *Chem. Zbl.* II. 2489.

Tindimnik, V.S., S.E. Funk, I.V. Sabinskaja. 1951. Kvoprosu o terapevticeskih svojstvah cajnogo griba. *Terapevticeskif Archiv* 23 (1) 85-87. (The question of the therapeutic vinegar bacteria therapeutic quality of the tea mushroom. Referat: Rentz, N. 1951)

Sass, E. Ju. 1952. O cajnom gribe. *Aptecnoje delo* (Moskva) (5) 41-42. (Tea mushroom.)

Buu-H oi, N.P., and A.R. Ratsimamanga. 1953. Kojic acid, active principal in the *Aspergillus flavus oryzae* culture. C.R. Acad. Sci. (Paris) 286, 341-343.

Anonymous. 1955. Kombucha. In: Der grosse Brockhaus, Bd. 16, 498. Wiesbaden: F.A. Brockhaus. 16. Aufl. p. 754.

Konovalov, I.N. and M.N. Semenova. 1955. K. Fiziologii "Cainogo gribva", *Bot. Zurnal* (Moskva) 40, 567-570. (The Physiology of the Tea mushroom.)

Prod'hom G. 1955. Mushroom of charity. *Bull. romand Mucolog.* (Lausanne) Dec., 1955.

Anonymous. 1956. Scientific Research at the Natural History Museum. 31. London: The trustees of the British Museum. p. 46.

Radu, A. 1956. Ciuperca de ceai. *Farmacia, Rev. Soc. Stintelor Med.* (Bucurest) 4, (4) 306-313. (Der Teepilz).

Strubin, M. 1956. Mushroom of charity. *Bull. romand Mycolog.* (Lausanne). Feb.

Flück, V. and E. Steinegger. 1957. A new yeast from the tea mushroom. *Sci. pharm.* 25, 43-44.

Flück, V. and E. Steinegger. 1957. Things worth knowing about the tea mushroom. Referat: Steiger, K.E. and Steinegger, E. The tea mushroom. *Osterr. Apoth.-Zig.* 11 (47) 580, 582-583.

Steiger, K.E. and E. Steinegger. 1957. The tea mushroom. (Sammel-referat.) *Pharm. Acta Helv.* 32, 133-154. (Referat: Sp. 1957).

Resources

Laurel Farms
P.O. Box 7405
Studio City, CA 91614
(310) 289-4372

Pronatura
6211-A West Howard
Niles, IL 60714
(708) 588-0900

Kombucha King International
P.O. Box 44203
Phoenix, AZ 85064
(602) 263-0792

For Other Medicinal Mushrooms (reishi, shiitake, etc):

Fungi Perfecti
P.O. Box 7634
Olympia, WA 98507
(206) 426-9292

Maitake Products
P.O. Box 1354
Paramas, NJ 07653
(800) 747-7418

North American Reishi Ltd.
Box 1780
Gibsons, B.C.
CANADA V0N 1V0
(604) 886-7799

Western Biologicals
Box 283
Alder Grove, B.C.
CANADA V0X 1A0
(604) 856-3339

For complete information on this subject, please see Christopher Hobbs' book, *Medicinal Mushrooms*, also available from the sources above.